What an
Pap Smear Means

Dedication

To all women who have ever had an abnormal Pap smear result.

What an Abnormal Pap Smear Means

Margaret Wilson, RN, RM

HILL OF CONTENT
Melbourne

First published in Australia 1994
by Hill of Content Publishing Company Pty Ltd
86 Bourke Street
Melbourne 3000 Australia

Figures and cover illustrated by Alison Scarfe
Designed and edited by Helen Burnett
Cover designed by Kimberley Wilson and Helen Burnett

Printed in Australia by
Australian Print Group Maryborough Victoria

National Library of Australia
Cataloguing-Publication data

Wilson, Margaret, 1956 Apr 1 —
        Living for Tomorrow—a positive approach to the
        treatment of cervical cancer
        What an Abnormal Pap Smear Means

Includes index

ISBN 0 85572 243 6

1. Pap test   2. Cancer—Diagnosis   3. Cancer—Treatment

Title

614 5999

Foreword

There has been a growing awareness in recent times, not only of the need for regular Pap smear tests, but of the need for women to fully understand what their smear results actually mean and to query those results if abnormal symptoms persist.

Until Margaret wrote *"Living for Tomorrow—*a positive approach to the treatment of cervical cancer"*, available literature focussed on advanced medical technology and medical personnel, seemingly overlooking the people at the very heart — women. In that book Margaret addressed all those areas pertaining to cervical cancer which women with this disease, needed to know in their fight for their future.

As a result of writing *"Living for Tomorrow"*, Margaret decided that a lot of the information contained in it needed to be re-presented so that it could become available to **all** women who are sexually active.

This book, *"What an Abnormal Pap Smear Means"*, is presented in the same easy to read style as the first book. She carefully and accurately describes the various gradations of cervical cell abnormalities, as well as exploring the various causes and probable treatments. Again, she poses and answers questions which may be considered too trivial or embarrassing to ask a doctor; and again, she provides a series of questions she considers essential that a doctor should be asked if a woman is presented with an abnormal Pap smear result.

Margaret should be congratulated once again, on bringing easily understood information within the grasp of all women.

Professor Robert S Planner
University of Melbourne
Mercy Hospital for Women
Melbourne

Acknowledgements

In February 1994, the release of the first book in my "*Living for Tomorrow*" series, signalled my personal and professional commitment to women's health in our society — a commitment based on my belief that a book series of this nature was not only necessary, but essential to women's clear understanding of particular health issues which may affect them personally.

Whilst this book specifically addresses the meaning of abnormal Pap smear results, it must, because of this, also duplicate sections of "*Living for Tomorrow*".

My sincere thanks to Professor Robert Planner, who yet again, in his busy schedule, painstakingly reviewed this manuscript with expertise, valuable advice and enthusiasm.

My special and sincere thanks to Dr Andrew Magennis and Helen Burnett for their dynamic enthusiasm, support and advice; who always fuel my steadfast determination and focussed thinking; and again to Helen for her design and editing, as well as for typing part of the manuscript. My thanks also to Christine Healy for her hard work in contributing so much to the typing of the manuscript.

To Alison Scarfe, the illustrator of my previous book, my thanks and appreciation for her superb line drawings thoughout the book.

My thanks to the various women in the community with whom I spoke and who shared with me their feelings and experiences of receiving an abnormal Pap smear, through to the investigative and treatment procedures they underwent.

My thanks to Professor Norman Beischer, Chairman, Department of Obstetrics and Gynaecology, University of Melbourne for granting me permission to use the photographs from the *Illustrated Text Book of Gynaecology*, 1990, 2nd Edition (E Mackay, N Beischer, R Pepperell, C Wood) and a selection of photographs from the University of Melbourne and Mercy Hospital for Women, Melbourne; and to Joseph Shramp for his valuable assistance in locating these photographs.

To Michelle Anderson for her support and belief in the importance of books on women's health issues, my thanks.

To Brian Ward of Brian Ward & Partners, my sincere thanks for his valuable advice and support.

Again, my special love and thanks to my husband and children for their patience, understanding, love and support during the writing of both books. To my friends and family for support and encouragement — Marilyn, Denise, Noeline, Nicci, Elizabeth, my sister Susie, my father and his wife Lencie, my mother and always ... Rosemary.

Table of Contents

Page

Introduction

During the last three years in Australia, the recognition of womens' health issues at a Federal level has seen the development of "The Organised Approach to Preventing Cancer of the Cervix" and the subsequent increasing awareness amongst women who have ever been sexually active between the ages of 18 to 70, of the importance of regular two-yearly Pap smear tests.

Whilst this is a notable achievement in the recognition and development of preventative womens' health, it is unfortunate that there is little detailed information available to women when their Pap smear test returns a "positive" or "abnormal" result.

Each year, approximately two million women in Australia have a Pap smear test and it is estimated that as many as 250,000 **could** be abnormal. It is not **known** exactly how many women have an abnormal Pap smear result, because Victoria and Western Australia are the only States in Australia which have a Pap Smear Registry, with New South Wales intending to commence a registry in 1994. Despite such an anomaly in the system, increasing comment is emerging from health care workers, both anecdotal and observational, that an abnormal Pap smear result can cause considerable anxiety in women. Indeed, women often do not understand what an abnormal Pap smear result means or why and how the development of abnormal cells of the cervix occur.

For too many women, an abnormal Pap smear result for the first time, can raise many fears and concerns; most often fear of cancer, fear of loss of reproductive ability, fear of changes to sexual function, fear of investigative medical procedures and treatment, or fear of the unknown.

1

Many of these fears are often unspoken and yet they can remain uppermost in a woman's mind for some time: often relieved only when the opportunity to discuss their concerns and receive accurate information occurs.

It is still an unfortunate reality that today in the 1990s the information available and provided by health care workers to women who have had an abnormal Pap smear result is in general not adequate and therefore women are unable to have an informed discussion on the meaning of their abnormal Pap smear test result.

It is therefore vital that, in addition to discussion with your doctor, you also have access to written information on what an abnormal Pap smear result means — including its causes — as well as possible investigative medical procedures which should occur.

This book is written essentially to provide this and other accurate information in order to allay any misconceptions, anxiety or concerns you may be experiencing at this time; but most of all to restore some normality to how you may be feeling. Whilst I do not attempt to provide all the answers, this book is written in the hope that it provides a baseline for further informed discussion between you and your doctor; a discussion where you have the right to ask questions and receive answers which you understand and to seek a second opinion from another doctor if you have doubts. Essential to your health, well-being and peace of mind, this book is written for you.

An abnormal Pap smear result can provoke feelings of anxiety and fear because you do not understand its meaning and significance — you may like to take the first step in resolving your feelings by reading this book. Over 90% of abnormalities of the cells of the cervix are **not** cancer; they are abnormal cells only and can occur for a variety of reasons.

I leave you with the thoughts of one lady:

I have had regular Pap smears for years and quite honestly did not ever consider that one day I would have a positive result. I knew such a result did not mean cancer, nevertheless I **was** concerned and worried.

My doctor explained the meaning of my positive Pap smear result and whilst I felt reassured, I did have some nagging doubts — particularly when he recommended that I see a gynaecologist for a colposcopic examination.

I had to wait six weeks for this examination and by the time I saw the gynaecologist I was quite upset; actually I was beside myself. At that stage I did not fully comprehend that the Pap smear test was meant as a "screening test" only and its result was not a diagnosis of anything!

Before I had the colposcopic examination I was absolutely petrified — but the colposcope was only a binocular microscope which looked at the cells of my cervix. This examination and a biopsy confirmed definite abnormalities of the cells of my cervix and these areas were treated by laser — as an outpatient — successfully!!

In retrospect I worried unnecessarily, because I did not understand what abnormal cells meant — I thought it was cancer!!! I now know differently.

One Woman's Comments

Margaret

PART I

Female Reproductive Organs and Location of the Cervix

There are many reasons for an abnormal Pap smear result and to understand such results it may be helpful for you to have an understanding of your female reproductive organs and the location of your cervix. Your reproductive organs are comprised of two ovaries, two fallopian tubes, a uterus, a cervix and a vagina — all located inside the pelvic area of your body.

The ovaries resemble large almonds in shape and size — approximately 3cms long and 2cms wide — and are located on each side of the pelvic area below the fallopian tubes. The ovaries produce female hormones — oestrogen and progesterone — and each ovary contains approximately 200,000 ova or egg cells.

The fallopian tubes are attached to the uterus, one on either side, and each month an egg is released from an ovary (they alternate monthly) and travels along the fallopian tube. If sperm reaches the egg in the fallopian tube during this time, fertilisation occurs and the fertilised egg moves along the tube and into the uterus where it embeds itself in the wall of the uterus and develops into an embryo and foetus, resulting in the birth of a child 40 weeks later. If fertilisation does not occur, the egg is shed each month in the form of menstruation (bleeding) from the vagina.

The uterus is a pear-shaped organ — approximately 8cms long and 6cms wide in the non-pregnant state — with the ability to enlarge enough to accommodate a growing foetus during pregnancy and then "shrink" back to its normal size after birth. The uterus has two main parts — the upper portion or "body" and a lower, narrow section — the cervix — which protrudes into the vagina.

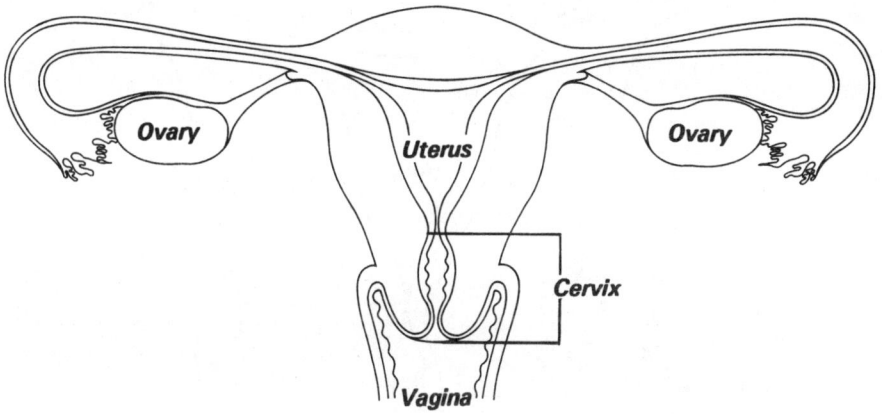

Figure 1—Female Reproductive Organs

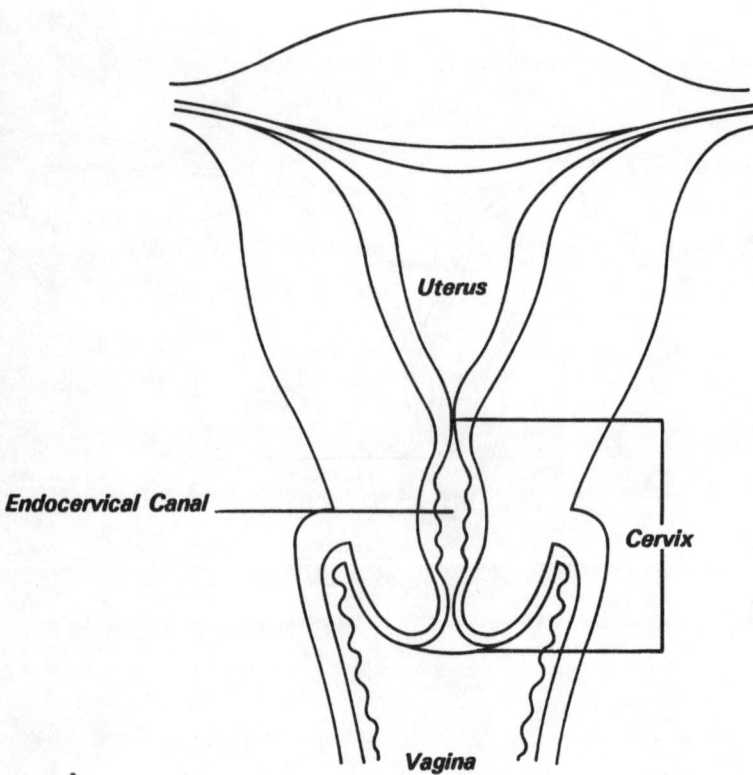

Figure 2—The Uterus and Cervix

Structure and Function of the Cervix

The cervix protrudes into the vagina and lies at the entrance to the uterus. Transversing the narrow section of the cervix is a canal called the endocervical canal which is approximately 2.5cms long. The entrance to this canal is called the external OS and it is this part of the cervix which protrudes into the vagina.

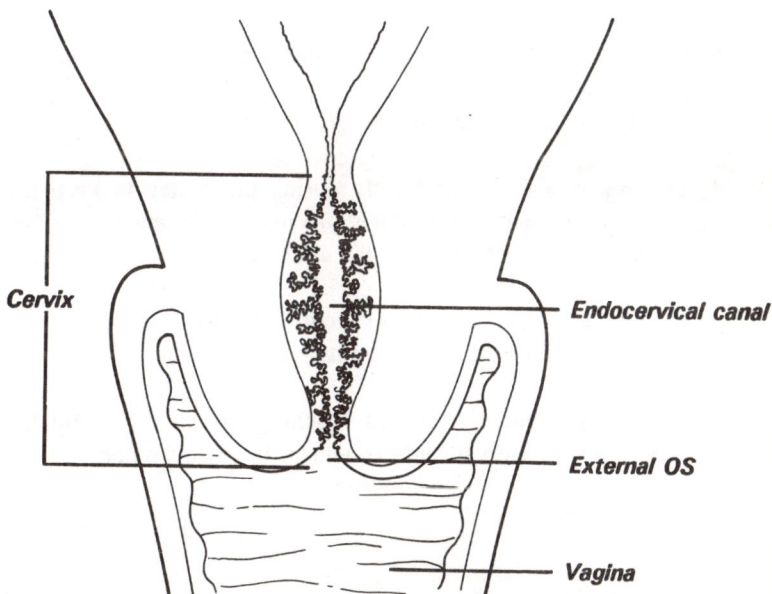

Figure 3—The Cervix

The vagina is composed of the same type of muscle as the uterus and has the ability to stretch, allowing the passage of a baby during birth. Following childbirth, the vagina then contracts to its normal size of 5-7cms long.

The cervix plays an important and interesting function in its role as part of the reproductive organs—

- It has an abundant blood supply, hence the bleeding which often occurs when cervical cancer is present and becomes invasive.

- The cells of the endocervical canal produce mucus which increases during sexual arousal and is thought to assist the passage of sperm to the uterus. During sexual arousal, the vagina also "balloons" at the end near the cervix and increases its size dramatically, which may also assist the passage of sperm to the uterus.

- During pregnancy the cervix produces a thick mucus plug to occlude the cervical canal and thereby provide a barrier against infection to the uterus and the growing foetus.

- The cervix also closes tightly during pregnancy to keep the foetus in the uterus and dilates (opens) during labour to allow the passage of the baby from the uterus and through the vagina.

- Monthly menstrual blood loss occurs from the uterus and flows through the cervix and the vagina.

- During intercourse, repeated touching of the cervix by the penis, can increase sexual excitement in some women.

Cells of the Cervix

Our body is composed of many different types of cells which perform specific functions. The cervix and vagina are composed of two different types of cells: the cells which line the endocervical canal are called **columnar** cells and these are the cells which produce mucus; the cells which line the vagina are called **squamous** cells. Columnar cells in the endocervical canal form a single column of cells side by side, whereas squamous cells in the vagina lie in several layers and are flat, like our skin.

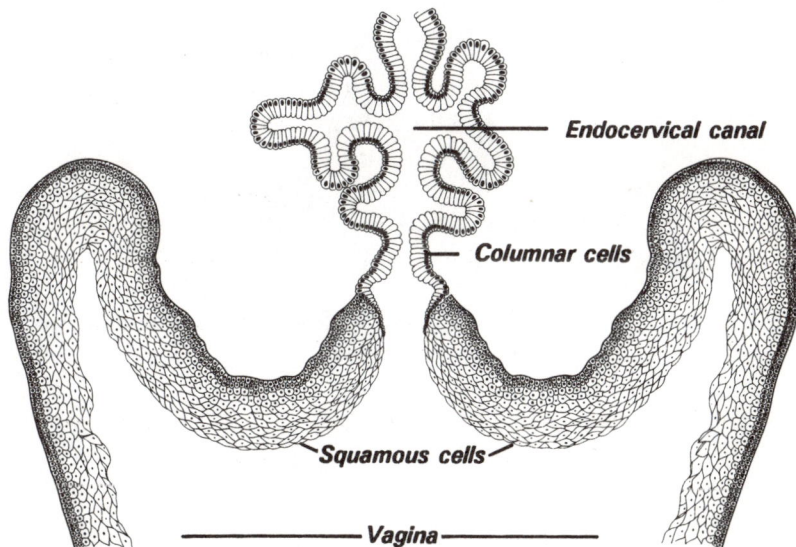

Endocervical canal

Columnar cells

Squamous cells

Vagina

Figure 4— The position of normal squamous and columnar cells of the cervix

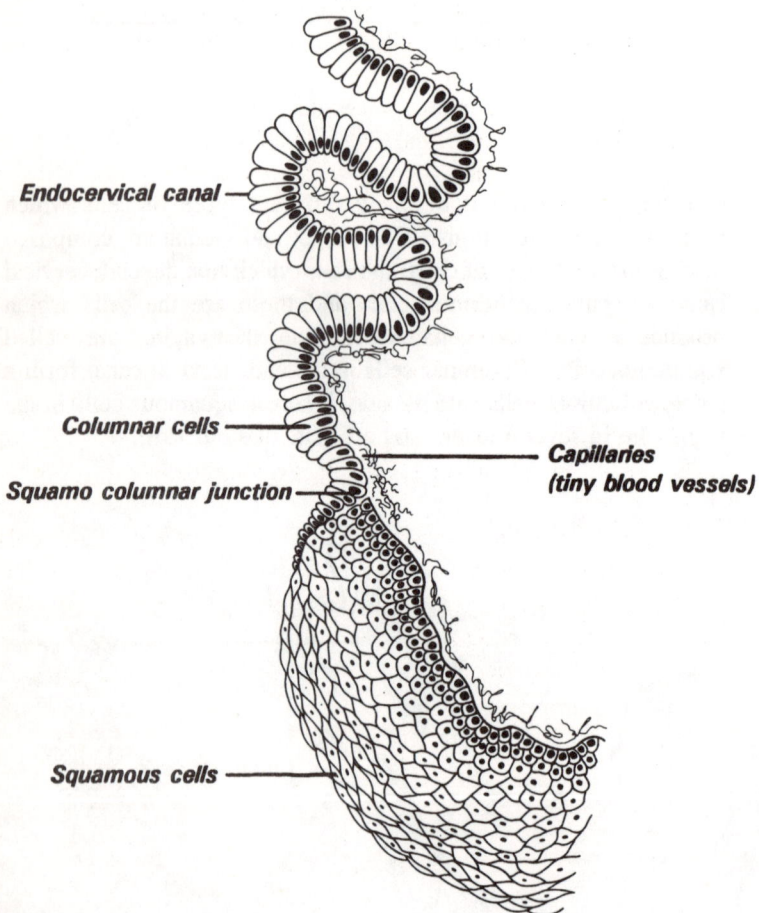

Figure 5—Transformation Zone

*The area where the squamous cells of the cervix
meet the columnar cells of the endocervical canal*

The area where the squamous cells of the outer part of the cervix (which protrude into the vagina) and the columnar cells in the endocervical canal meet is called the **squamo-columnar junction** (squamous cells-columnar cells) or the **transformation zone**.

Before puberty and after menopause (when no oestrogen is produced by the ovaries), the transformation zone is located inside the alkaline environment of the endocervical canal, not far from the external OS.

When the ovaries start to function at puberty, and oestrogen is produced, the endocervical canal everts into the acid environment of the vagina and the transformation zone is located on the ectocervix (the surface of the cervix and external OS). Exposure of the columnar cells (previously in the endocervical canal) to this acid environment in the vagina changes these cells into squamous cells; this change is normal and called **metaplasia**.

The transformation zone of the cervix changes constantly depending on the level of oestrogen in the body. At times, when oestrogen levels are higher (during adolescence and pregnancy), metaplasia is occurring rapidly and the transformation zone everts further into the ectocervix.

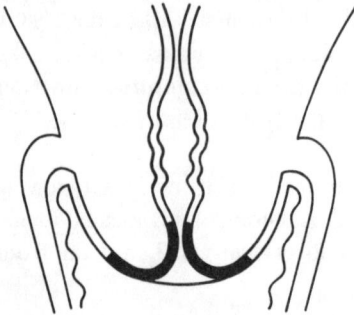

Transformation Zone during
puberty and pregnancy when
oestrogen levels are higher

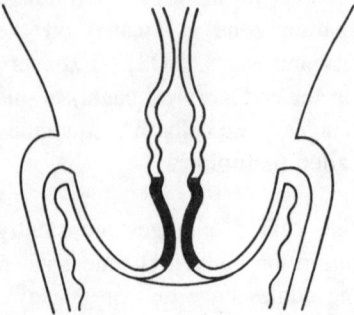

Transformation Zone during
reproductive life

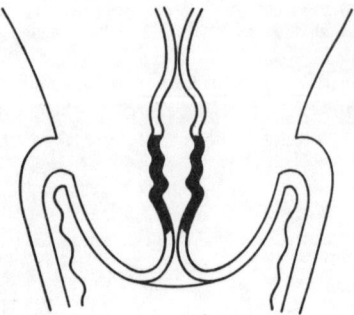

Transformation Zone before
puberty and after menopause
when oestrogen levels are low

Figure 6—Transformation Zone,
Endocervical Canal and Ectocervix

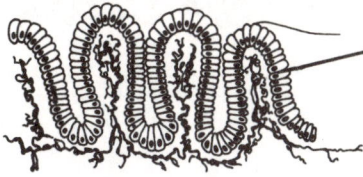

Columnar cells in the endocervical canal are exposed to the acid environment of the vagina which constantly changes these cells into squamous cells

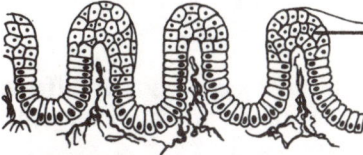

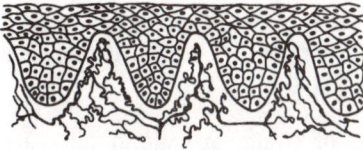

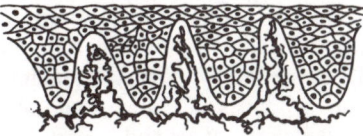

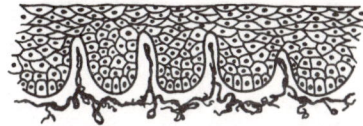

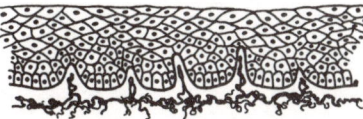

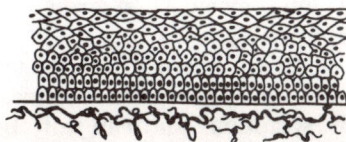

Squamous cells

Figure 7—
Transformation Zone
Metaplasia

Reproduced from
"The Atlas of Colposcopy"
3rd Edition, 1982
A Stafl, P Kolstad;
with permission of
Professor A Stafl

Abnormal Cells of the Cervix

As we have seen, our body is made up of a collection of different cells and the two types of cells in the cervix are called squamous and columnar.

There are three phases in the life cycle of a normal cell: it evolves, develops and matures to perform its useful function and then dies, to be replaced by a new cell.

Metaplasia, the normal changing of columnar cells to squamous cells at the transformation zone, occurs constantly. When new cells are required the columnar cells or squamous cells divide in two, and these then divide again, and again, until the required number of new cells is achieved. Sometimes a normal squamous cell or a normal columnar cell produces an abnormal cell. Abnormal cells are immature or undeveloped cells and they in turn may produce more immature cells. The nucleus (the important growth centre of a cell), generally small, is quite large in an immature cell.

Abnormal cells of the cervix — Cervical Intra-epithelial Neoplasia — are referred to as CIN for short, or sometimes as cervical dysplasia.

C = Cervix
I   = Intra-epithelial (or within the skin)
N = Neoplasia (or change in the cells)

The degree of abnormality present in the cells is classified as CIN 1, 2 or 3; dysplasia is classified as mild, moderate or severe.

The purpose of a Pap smear is to detect abnormal cells of the cervix, which if **undetected** or **untreated**, can progress to cervical cancer. **CIN causes no signs or symptoms and can only be detected by a Pap smear.**

CIN 1 (Mild Dysplasia)

This is characterised by a few immature cells amongst mostly mature cells. The abnormal cells extend through one-third of the thickness of the epithelium or cervical skin.

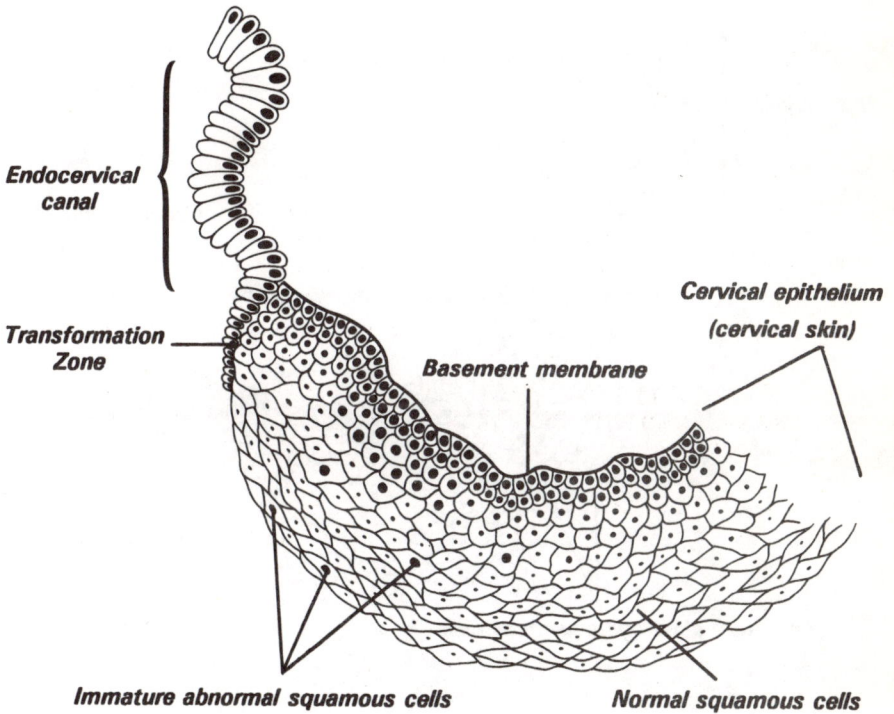

Figure 8—CIN 1 (Mild Dysplasia)

CIN 2 (Moderate Dysplasia)

This is characterised by increasing numbers of immature cells. These cells are pre-cancerous and if not removed can progress to carcinoma insitu or invasive cancer. Abnormal cells now involve up to half the thickness of the epithelium or cervical skin.

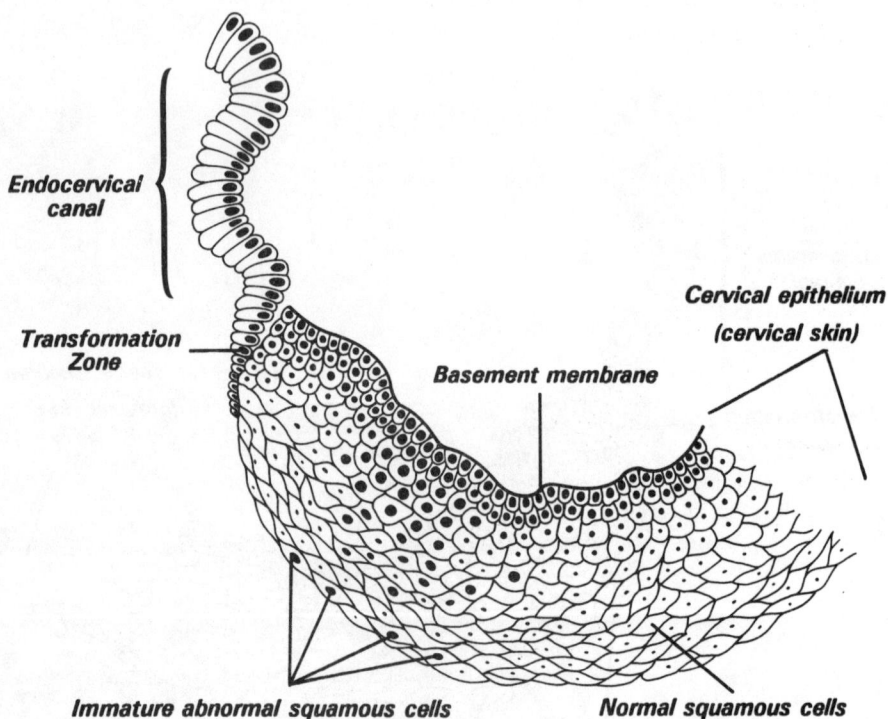

Figure 9—CIN 2 (Moderate Dysplasia)

CIN 3 (Severe Dysplasia)

Previously known as carcinoma insitu, this Stage, whilst it sounds ominous, can be effectively treated. It is characterised by large numbers of immature cells. There are few normal cells present at this Stage and although the abnormal cells are almost cancerous in appearance, they remain confined within the epithelium or cervical skin. While they do not have the capacity to invade blood and lymph vessels or spread, urgent and immediate investigation and treatment is required.

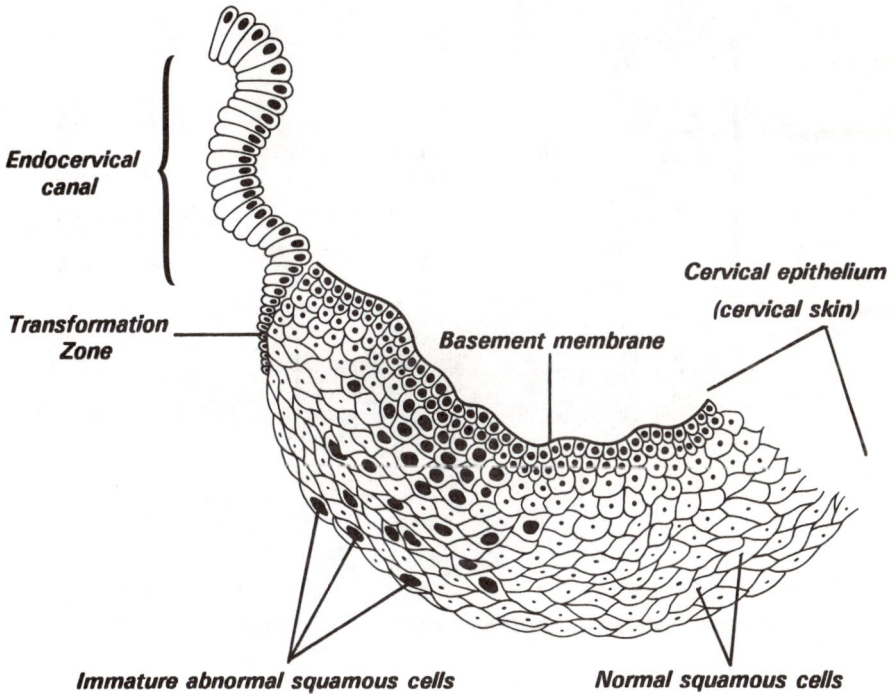

Figure 10—CIN 3 (Severe Dysplasia)
(Previously known as Carcinoma Insitu)

Micro-Invasive Carcinoma

The cells are malignant (cancerous) and have broken through the basement membrane invading to a depth of up to 3mm. They have not invaded blood or lymph vessels, but if not adequately treated will both invade deeper into the cervix as well as develop the ability to spread to the lymph nodes. Treatment can be a cone biopsy or simple hysterectomy.

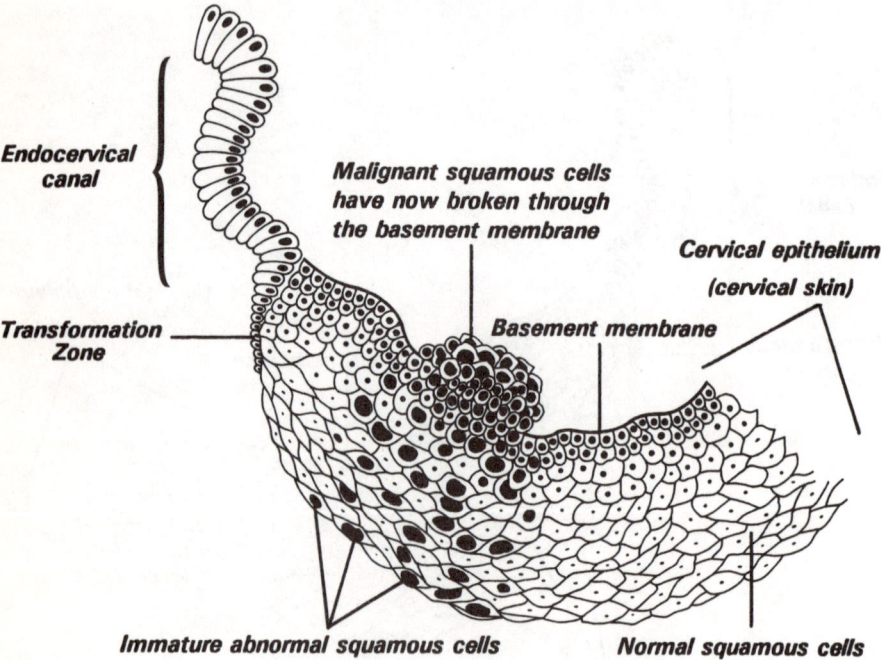

Figure 11—Micro-Invasive Carcinoma

Invasive Squamous Cell Carcinoma

(or Adeno Carcinoma) (Carcinoma of the columnar cells).

This is characterised by malignant cells invading the deep tissues of the cervix and is more likely to develop local spread to the vagina or secondary spread to pelvic lymph nodes by invading and traversing lymphatic vessels. The incidence of spread to these other sites is dependent upon a number of factors, such as the size and the type of cancer. Invasive cancer may also be microscopic (not visible to the naked eye) or obvious as either an ulcer or growth on the cervix. Early invasive cancer confined to the cervix can generally be successfully treated.

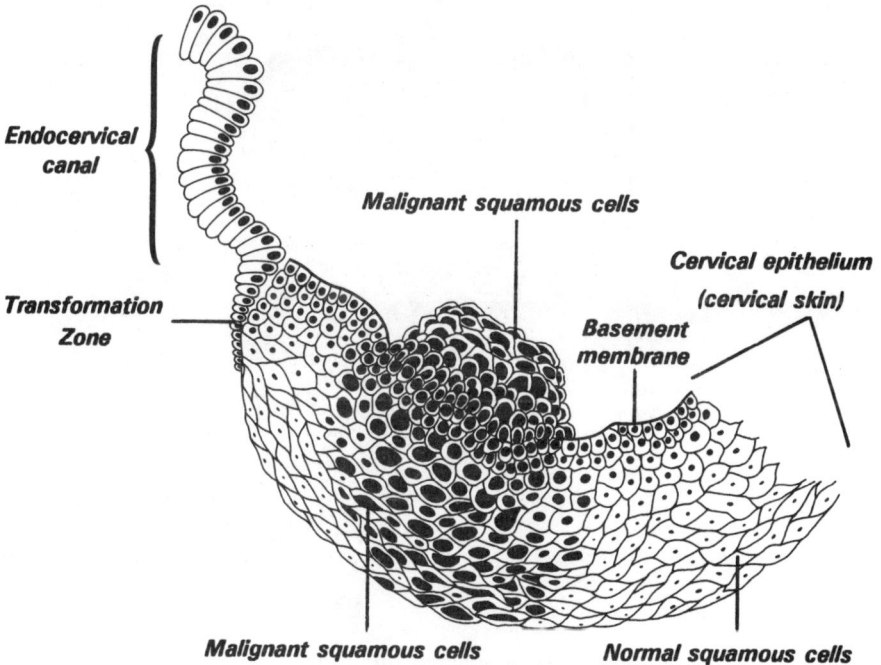

Endocervical canal

Malignant squamous cells

Cervical epithelium (cervical skin)

Transformation Zone

Basement membrane

Malignant squamous cells

Normal squamous cells

Figure 12—Invasive Squamous Cell Carcinoma

Not all abnormal cells of the cervix will progress to malignant cancer cells. Some abnormal cells will spontaneously revert to normal, others will not. As yet, doctors are unable to predict whose cells will progress to cancer and whose will revert to normal. It is for this reason that CIN is closely observed or treated. There is also no way of determining how long CIN is present before it can progress to cancer — in some women it may be months — in others, years.

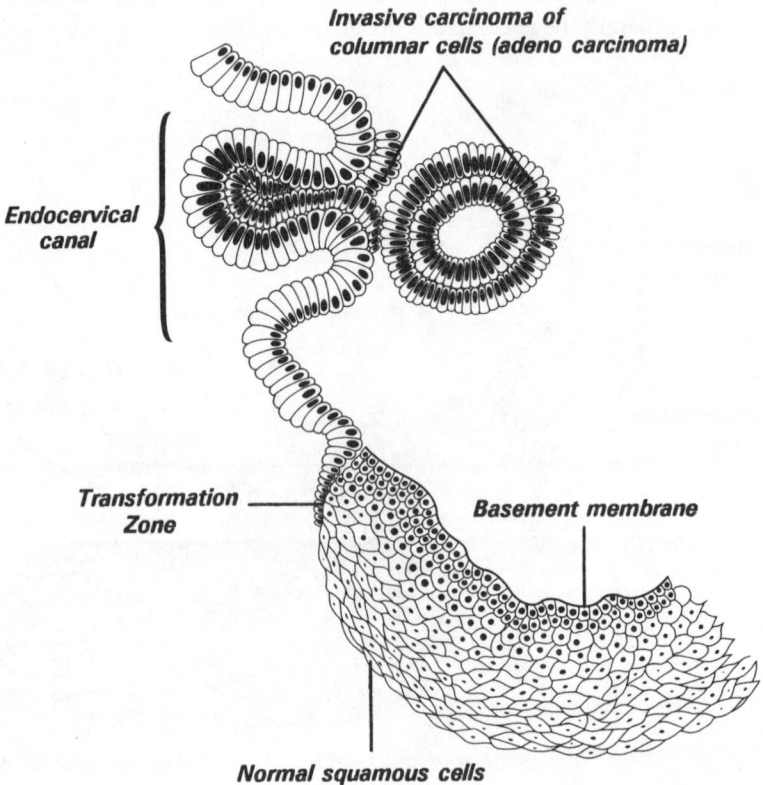

Figure 13—Invasive Adeno Carcinoma

PART II

What Causes Abnormal Cells of the Cervix?

As we have already seen, there are three phases in the life cycle of a normal cell: it evolves, develops and matures to perform its useful function, and then dies to be replaced by a new cell.

When new cells are required, for example in the cervix, the columnar cells and squamous cells of the cervix divide in two and then divide again and again until the required number of new cells is achieved. Sometimes a normal squamous cell or a normal columnar cell produces an abnormal cell. Abnormal cells are immature or under-developed cells and they in turn may produce more immature cells.

Why? The exact reason has yet to be established. However, to date, what is known from extensive medical studies, is that abnormal cells of the cervix generally occur in women who have been sexually active. As we already know, if abnormal cells (CIN) are not detected through regular Pap smears and then treated, they may develop into cancerous cells.

It is also known that abnormal cells of the cervix and cervical cancer occur **rarely** in women who have never had sexual intercourse — for example nuns. It would therefore seem from medical evidence to date, that a clear relationship between sexual intercourse and the development of abnormal cells of the cervix does exist. There are also several theories as to how the link between intercourse and the development of abnormal cells may occur.

There are no less than six to ten possible pre-disposing causes to the development of abnormal cells of the cervix and probably many more which have yet to be identified and the following are but a few:

• *Human Papilloma Virus (HPV) — Wart Virus*

The exact incidence of HPV is unknown, but it is estimated that up to 60% of women have HPV, commonly known as the wart virus. Recent research has revealed that over 90% of women who have CIN also have HPV Types 16 or 18 (of the 70+ types of wart virus known), identified on biopsy of their abnormal or malignant cervical cells. Less common types associated with abnormal cells are HPV Types 31, 33, 35 and 37.

The wart virus may be found in the cervix, vagina and external vulva; there may be no symptoms and its presence detected only on a Pap smear test. It appears, therefore, that the wart virus could be implicated in the development of abnormal cells of the cervix, although many women who have **not** had intercourse have the wart virus in their genital tract (cervix, vagina).

Research into HPV is continuing and it is thought that HPV **may** be transmitted during intercourse from one person who has the virus to another who does not; or even that the virus is always present.

Researchers are currently working on a vaccination in an effort to prevent the development of the wart virus.

Some women may develop genital warts (Types 6 and/or 11) where small visible warts are obvious on the external genital area and whilst embarrassing, they virtually never progress to cancer. Over 60% of women with genital warts respond successfully to one or two local treatments; 20% may require several treatments and a periodic review; and the remaining 20% will find the warts spontaneously regress without treatment.

The idea that genital warts and promiscuity go hand-in-hand is unproven. If it were the case then 60% of the female population would be labelled promiscuous and from independent studies done throughout the world, this is definitely not true.

> When I developed genital warts I was referred to a gynaecologist for localised treatment. I felt very embarrassed and vulnerable.
>
> After the treatment was completed the doctor said to me: "I bet you won't sleep with anyone without using a condom now!"
>
> I felt very humiliated by such a harsh judgmental and ignorant remark — I have only had one partner.

One Woman's Comments

• *Herpes Virus*

The herpes virus, which presents as genital herpes, is sexually transmitted and is also evident in some women who develop abnormal cells of the cervix. Treatment for genital herpes is symptomatic. Lesions near the entrance to the vagina are evident as ulcers or blisters.

The wart virus and herpes virus may be sexually transmitted by a man to a woman who did not have these viruses previously and therefore pre-dispose the development of abnormal cells of the cervix.

• *Partner's Occupation*

In 1978, BL Read, PW French and A Singer identified "basic proteins" found in high quantities in the sperm of some men. It was established that this affected cells of the cervix causing abnormalities and cervical cancer and seemed to be related to the occupation and social class of the husbands whose wives developed cervical cancer.

The **exact** relationship between economic class and cervical cancer has not been clearly identified. It has been hypothesised that partners with occupations which involve working with dust, oil or chemicals may absorb them into the body, hence the increase in "basic protein" found in sperm.

In 1981, JD Buckley and colleagues conducted a study of the husbands of women with dysplasia and cervical cancer. They found that women were at higher risk if their husbands had 15 or more partners outside marriage.

• *Smoking*

Research into smoking and cervical cancer has concluded that smoking increases the risk of developing cervical cancer. This occurs because the carcinogens in cigarettes are absorbed into the body and excreted in cervical mucus, lowering the immunity of the cells of the cervix. Local defence cells of the cervix, called Langerhans Cells, are found to be absent in smokers.

• *Oral Contraceptives*

There is no clear evidence to link the pill with cancer. There was some hypotheses, years ago, that the pill caused cervical cell abnormality. Because women did not have to worry about falling pregnant it was hypothesised that they were therefore more likely to have several sexual partners as a result.

• *Sexual Partners*

The relationship between squamous cell carcinoma of the cervix and the number of sexual partners women have had is well documented in medical literature. In Buckley's study he found that the risk of developing cervical cancer increased with the number of sexual partners, ie more than seven, but once again the exact **cause** of the increased risk is not clear.

• *Age of Sexual Intercourse*

The cervix is more vulnerable at or around puberty because of the rapid onset of columnar cells transforming to squamous cells at the transformation zone. Also, since few teenagers are likely to remain with one partner at this experimental age of their sexuality, it is likely that they may have several partners, which further increases the risk of the development of abnormal cells on their still maturing cervix, which is more vulnerable to the development of abnormal cells of the cervix.

It is clear that any woman who has sexual intercourse is at risk. However, there are many women who develop abnormal cells of the cervix who have only had one partner, their partner has only had one partner, they do not smoke, they do not have the wart virus and are in a middle to upper social and occupational class.

Many women fear they will be judged promiscuous by friends, family and health professionals and some will be made to feel guilty about their own sexuality if they have had more than one partner. Some are quick to defend their sexual history and may feel they have to justify their sexual behaviour, be it with one or more partners, to stop their own fear that others will presume they "slept around". This can also cause a problem in marriages if cervical cancer is diagnosed, where partners may "blame" each other for past sexual histories which may be non-existent.

Apart from intercourse, a definite cause has not been established; and even then the **reason** intercourse causes abnormal cells of the cervix and cancer of the cervix is not clear. It is all hypothesis and speculation. Unfortunately for the woman who develops CIN or cervical cancer, the hypothetical cause has become an accepted **fact** in society.

In 1981 Richardson and Lyon conducted a study of women with CIN where one group of women were told to use condoms and the second group did not. The study was abandoned after it was discovered that the women whose partners used condoms had a significant regression in the presence of CIN. However, there were several weaknesses to this study including a lack of controls.

Of course, with the implication that sex causes CIN, many women may be afraid that it will develop again.

In 1990, Thomas *et al* at the Royal Women's Hospital, Brisbane conducted a controlled study of 44 women with CIN 1, whereby for six months the partners of 24 women used condoms during intercourse and 20 did not. They concluded that "contrary to the declaration of Richardson & Lyon, the therapeutic value of the condom is not obvious", with a final comment that there is no place for condoms alone in the treatment of CIN.

Pap Smear Tests

The role of the Pap smear test is to identify abnormal or pre-cancerous changes in the cells of the cervix which, if undetected or untreated, may progress to cervical cancer. As we have seen, abnormal cells of the cervix are referred to as CIN or dysplasia and cause no signs or symptoms.

The Pap smear test is named after Dr George Papanicolaou who developed it in the 1920s. Its true value was not recognised until 20 years later and today, in 1994, it remains the only screening test available worldwide which can detect abnormal cells before they become cancerous. The Pap smear is indeed unique for this reason.

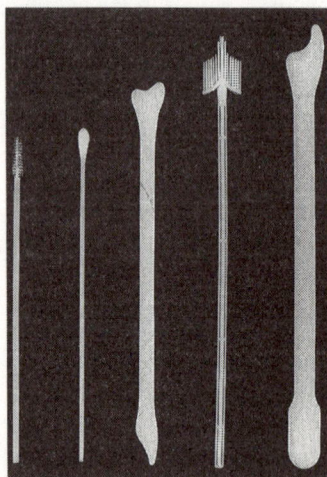

Figure 14—Photograph of Instruments for Pap Smear Examinations
Photograph courtesy of Professor N Beischer from
The Illustrated Book of Gynaecology, 1990, 2nd edition

How is a Pap Smear Test Taken?

You will be required to remove all clothing from your waist down and will be asked to lie on your back on an examination couch with a blanket or similar covering over you.

With your knees bent and parted but with your ankles together, the doctor or nurse will gently insert a plastic or metal speculum into your vagina, so that the walls of the vagina are parted (they normally lie in opposition) and the cervix can be visualised. Some doctors may place you in another position where you lie on your side with your knees drawn up toward your chest.

A sample of the squamous and columnar cells of the transformation zone of the cervix is taken using a small wooden spatula. The cells of the endocervical canal (columnar cells) are also sampled using a tiny brush not unlike a mascara brush. This procedure takes only a few minutes and at the most is slightly uncomfortable, but not painful. You can then dress.

> Remember to ring your doctor or health centre for the results in a week. It is best to have a Pap smear test two weeks after your period and not during the time you are menstruating.

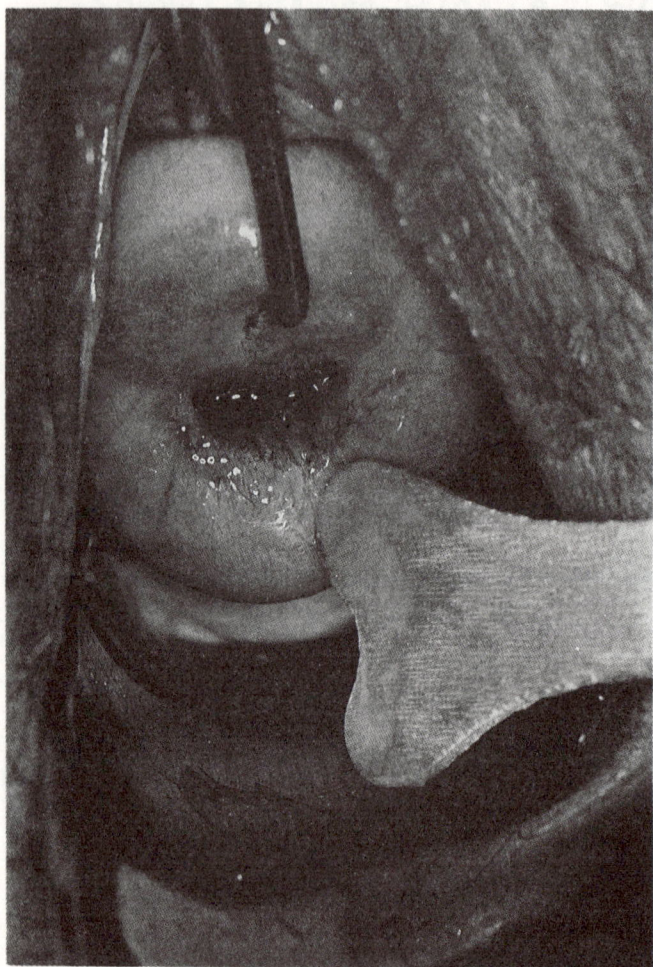

Figure 15—Photograph of the Cervix

A wooden spatula is used to sample the cells of the cervix during a Pap smear test. Note that the forceps holding the cervix are not used when a Pap smear test is taken. The photograph is courtesy of Professor N Beischer, University of Melbourne, Department of Obstetrics and Gynaecology, Mercy Hospital for Women, Melbourne.

When you ring for the results of your Pap smear test, always check that endocervical and squamous cells have been identified on your pathology report. Both endocervical and squamous cells are essential components of a successfully taken Pap smear.

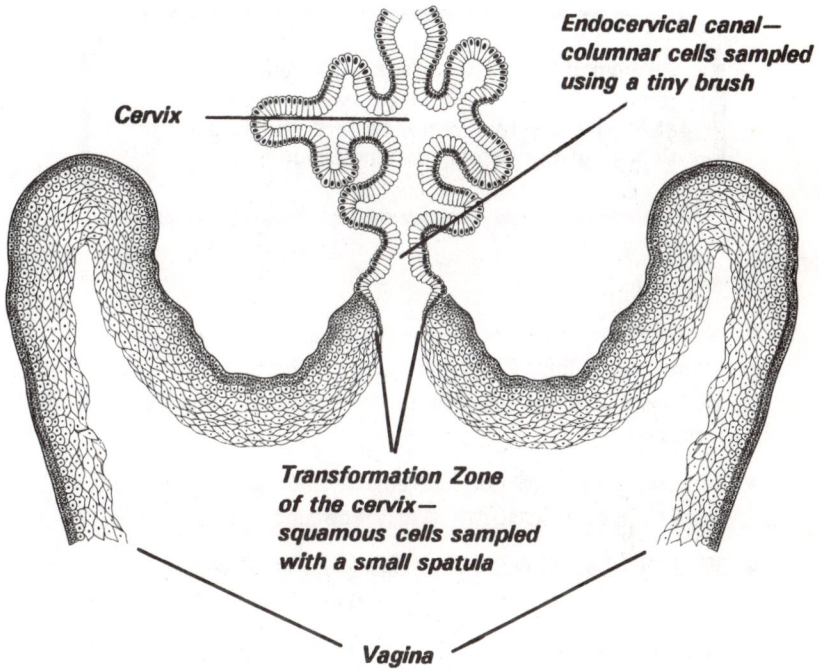

Figure 16—Diagram of cells of the Endocervical Canal and Transformation Zone, sampled during a Pap smear test

Who Should Have a Pap Smear Test?

Screening for cervical cancer by Pap smear has been available in Australia for over 30 years, yet until 1988, there had not been adequate public education on the necessity for regular Pap smears for all women who have ever been sexually active.

> **All women who have had sexual intercourse** between the ages of 18 and 70 should have a Pap smear test at least every two years, as recommended by the College of Gynaecologists and Obstetricians.

Be aware that:

- Any female who becomes sexually active should have a Pap smear test within 12 months of first intercourse — including teenagers. Abnormal cells of the cervix can and do occur in teenagers.

- Women who have not had sexual intercourse for years still need to have at least two-yearly Pap smear tests.

- Women who are post-menopausal and no longer have periods should still have at least two-yearly Pap smear tests.

- Women who have had a hysterectomy do not need Pap smear tests unless their surgery was performed for cancer of the cervix or for CIN. Women who have had endometrial ablation (surgical removal of the lining of the uterus) and women who have had sub-total hysterectomies (where the cervix is retained) still need to have regular Pap smear tests because the cervix has not been removed. However, annual pelvic examinations and general check-ups are advisable, as the risk of ovarian and breast cancer increases with age.

Vaginal Discharge

Beware of persistent unexplained vaginal discharge — for example a constant clear watery discharge, or blood-stained discharge — and see your doctor for a Pap smear test and further investigation, irrespective of the smear result..

Vaginal Bleeding

- Bleeding after intercourse
- Irregular bleeding or spotting
- Bleeding after menopause

Abnormal symptoms such as these need investigation, irrespective of a Pap smear result, ie a negative Pap smear does not cancel abnormal symptoms.

Ask for a referral to a gynaecologist or gynaecologist-oncologist for further investigation of these symptons

I was successfully treated for genital warts two years ago and was told that the wart virus was present in the cells of my cervix, but no other abnormalities.

A few months ago I noticed slight spotting after intercourse and have since split up with my boyfriend. Finally, after talking about it with a friend, I decided to have a Pap smear test.

After the Pap smear test was taken, I bled profusely — there was a large gush of blood immediately. I was quite concerned because my period was not due for another two weeks. When I questioned my doctor about this, no explanation was given.

I have just received the results of my Pap smear and it was normal. Again, I questioned my doctor about the bleeding when my Pap test was taken, but feel I was "fobbed off".

I spoke to my girlfriend again and have now made an appointment at the dysplasia clinic where my genital warts were treated.

I'm scared stiff I have cancer of my cervix — I have never bled following a Pap smear test, ever.

One Woman's Comments

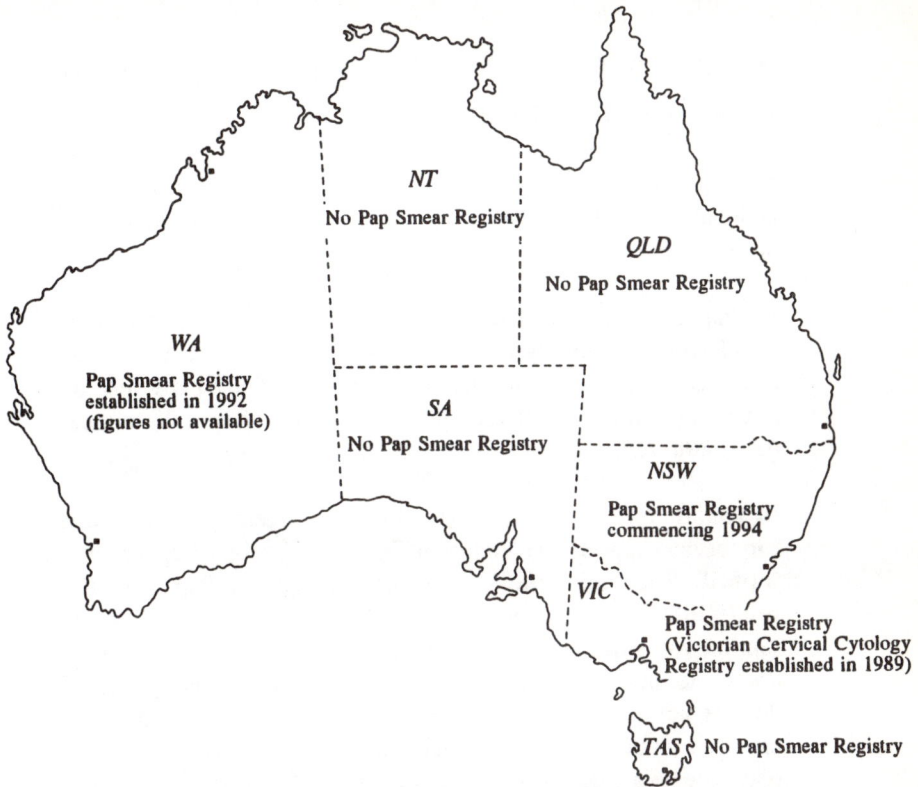

Map of Australia showing Pap Smear Registry status by state:

- **NT** — No Pap Smear Registry
- **QLD** — No Pap Smear Registry
- **WA** — Pap Smear Registry established in 1992 (figures not available)
- **SA** — No Pap Smear Registry
- **NSW** — Pap Smear Registry commencing 1994
- **VIC** — Pap Smear Registry (Victorian Cervical Cytology Registry established in 1989)
- **TAS** — No Pap Smear Registry

Victorian Cervical Cytology Registry Figures

Year	No of women screened by Pap smear	Histology / colposcopy results registered	No of women with CIN identified	No of women with micro-invasive cancer	No of women with cancer
1990	402,000	6,106	2,812	28	70
1991	498,000	7,644	3,437	36	143
1992	497,000	8,418	3,823	49	100
1993	523,000	8,859	4,060	29	116

Figure 17—Incidence of CIN in Victoria
Source—Victorian Cervical Cytology Registry
Statistical Reports 1990-1993

How Do I Remember to Have My Next Pap Smear Test?

In 1992, the Commonwealth Government initiated "The Organised Approach to Preventing Cancer of the Cervix" and developed a national preventative health program to inform and educate women on the importance of two-yearly Pap smear tests.

A "Pap Smear reminder card" was developed to last for ten years — all you do is simply mark the date when your next Pap smear test is due. If you do not have a free copy of this card you can obtain one from Medicare offices or via a free call number (008) 808 725.

In Victoria in 1990, in an effort to increase screening of all women for cervical cancer, the Victorian Cervical Cytology Registry was formed. The Register contains a confidential list of Pap smear test results of Victorian women and the Registry sends a letter to remind you when your next smear is due. You can request your doctor to include your name on the Register, although many doctors automatically seek your consent to do this. Letters are usually sent out three-yearly, but if an abnormality is evident, you may receive a letter of reminder for another Pap smear test earlier. There is also a Pap Test Registry in Western Australia and plans for a registry in New South Wales in 1994. It is expected that further registries will develop in other States of Australia at some later stage.

Why Don't Women Have Regular Pap Smear Tests?

The responsibility of helping to prevent cervical cancer by having regular Pap smear tests is twofold — individual responsibility and the responsibility of doctors to offer regular Pap smear tests and educate their female patients in the importance of the preventative role of having regular tests.

To many women, a Pap smear test provokes a feeling of embarrassment, intermingled with a sense of dread — embarrassment at the exposure of your genitals — your private female parts — to the doctor who is most often a male. There may be a feeling of dread that the doctor may be rough and insensitive to your emotional vulnerability at this time. There may be no conscious thought — it may be purely emotive — a feeling of unease — a baring of vulnerability. It is this emotion and the fallacy that it "cannot happen to me" which results in women not having regular Pap smear tests. Some women, on the offer of a Pap smear test by their doctor, will lie and say they are menstruating ("Phew! That was close! Got out of it again!").

> It is estimated that only 50% of the five million women between the ages of 18 and 70 in Australia have Pap smear tests every two years.

The incidence of CIN and cervical cancer seems to peak at ages 25-39 and 50-69. Women in the younger age group tend to be screened regularly. However, those in the 50-69 year age group are screened infrequently and are therefore more likely to progress from abnormal cells of the cervix to cervical cancer, because they are hesitant to have Pap smear tests.

Middle-aged women may be too embarrassed or hesitant to ask for a smear test, believing cervical cancer cannot happen to them; whilst others simply prefer not to know. Some of these women may have been screened in younger years as they raised their families simply by having frequent contact with their doctor because of children's illnesses and/or contraceptive advice. As children grow older and contraception advice is no longer sought, there may be a reduction in contact with their local doctor; hence many women of this age group are unlikely to present for a Pap smear test only.

Similarly, many women living in country areas may have poor access to Pap smear tests due to geographical location; or do not avail themselves of such a service by their family doctor, who may also be a family friend — which may be a source of embarrassment to the women.

Non-English speaking women and Aboriginal women are also at a disadvantage and may not present themselves for Pap smear tests because they are unaware that they exist, or do not realise the importance of this preventative health measure.

In October 1993, in an effort to increase cervical screening in the 50-69 year age group, the educational unit of the Anti-Cancer Council of Victoria undertook a three-year project of screening. Personalised letters of invitation to have a Pap smear test were sent out giving information on where to go to have a smear test done.

I hadn't had a Pap smear test for many years and am post-menopausal. Three years ago I developed bleeding after intercourse and saw my doctor promptly.

Following a colposcopic examination and punch biopsy, I was diagnosed as having very early cancer of the cervix. I had a hysterectomy and have never looked back.

If I had attended for regular Pap smear tests, abnormal cells of my cervix would have been detected and treated **before** they developed into cancer.

One Woman's Comments

Where can I have a Pap smear?

- **Your local Doctor**
- **Family Planning Clinic**
- **Well Women's Health Clinic**
- **Community Health Centre**
- **Women's Hospitals**

Analysis of Pap Smear Tests

The essential features required for the successful examination of a Pap smear are:

- A sufficient quantity of cells from the cervix.

- The presence of endocervical cells and squamous cells, which indicates that the cells of the endocervical canal and transformation zone have been sampled (see Figure 16).

Vaginal bleeding, infection or discharge can obscure the cells of the smear and if this occurs, it should be repeated. Subject to the sample being adequate, the cytopathologist will examine the smear for:

- Evidence of cell inflammation (infection) and metaplasia of columnar cells and squamous cells.

- The presence of abnormal cells (which may be due to infection, inflammation, hormone deficiency or of unknown significance).

- Evidence of CIN 1, 2 or 3 of squamous and columnar cells.

- The presence of HPV (Human Papilloma Virus).

Having examined the smear, the cytopathologist will then recommend what management he feels necessary. For example:

- Repeat the smear three-, six-, twelve-monthly or two-yearly.

- Repeat the smear after treating the infection present.

- A colposcopic examination or biopsy is recommended.

Results of Pap Smear Tests—What Do They Mean?

Following a Pap smear test, the results should be available at the doctor's surgery within a week and it is best to telephone for them and not rely on someone notifying you. It is always possible that a slip-up can occur between the surgery, computerised results or pathologist and although not intended, your result can be overlooked. Rely only on yourself and ensure you follow through and get your results. Your Pap smear test result may be negative, but as long as you do not have abnormal symptoms, remember to have another one in one or two years!

When you ring for the results of your Pap smear test, always check that both endocervical and squamous cells have been identified on your pathology report (see page 33).

If you telephone for the results of your Pap smear test and are told there are some abnormalities present, or the result is positive, **do not panic!** Ninety percent of abnormalities of cells of the cervix are **not** cancer; they are abnormal cells only and these can occur for a variety of reasons.

You should make an appointment to see your doctor, so that the nature of the abnormality can be explained to you.

- ***Inconclusive Result***
  This often reflects an inadequate sample of cells of the cervix having been taken and often a repeat smear will be recommended in four to eight weeks. If, however, a repeat smear of six months or longer is recommended, **query** it. It would be unwise to go beyond six weeks before you had a repeat smear and very unusual for a doctor to recommend you do so.

- ***Presence of Inflammation or Infection***
  Vaginal infections such as thrush or trichomonas can give a "positive" result. When smears reveal the presence of infection, you should be treated with the appropriate antibiotic and a repeat smear test performed four to six weeks after completion of the course of antibiotics. In the event that a second smear test continues to show the presence of inflammation, despite antibiotic treatment, ask for a referral to a gynaecologist. **Severe cell abnormalities, ie CIN 3, micro-invasive or invasive cancer, sometimes reveal themselves by indicating the presence of inflammation.**

- ***Post-menopausal Atrophy/Post-partum Atrophy***
  Lack of oestrogen can make interpretation difficult. Therefore a course of local oestrogen may be the recommended treatment by your doctor before repeating the smear test.

- ***Human Papilloma Virus (HPV)***
  The Human Papilloma Virus is often referred to as the Wart Virus and its presence in women's genital tracts is often a source of confusion, misunderstanding and anxiety to many.

  The exact incidence of HPV is unknown, but it is estimated that up to 60% of women have this virus in their genital tracts, ie the cervix, vagina and/or external genital organs (vulva, vaginal area), and over 70 types of HPV have been identified so far.

The presence of HPV may not cause any symptoms at all and only be detected on a Pap smear test. HPV in this situation produces **tiny microscopic** changes to the cells of the cervix, vagina or vulva. However, the majority of HPV changes to the cells are of **NO SIGNIFICANCE** and often spontaneously regress. When HPV is identified on a Pap smear, a repeat smear in six months is usually recommended and if HPV changes persist, investigation by colposcopy would be indicated to ascertain whether this has caused changes to the cells of the cervix (CIN, dysplasia).

> HPV Types 16 and 18, when given the **right conditions,** eg smoking, may produce CIN (dysplasia) of the cells of the cervix. It is for this reason that when these Types are identified on a Pap smear and CIN is evident, investigation with a colposcope is indicated.

Fears

It is not uncommon for women to experience fears that they will develop cervical cancer if the presence of HPV is identified on their Pap smear.

If you are in this situation and feel concerned and upset that you will develop cervical cancer **STOP WORRYING**.

> The majority of women with HPV **do not** develop CIN (dysplasia) or cervical cancer.

However, as we have already seen, **if** CIN does develop, this will be detected by regular Pap smear tests and treated easily — **before** cancer develops.

- ## *Genital Warts*
  The Human Papilloma Virus can also manifest as small visible warts, obvious on the external genital area, ie the vulva and around the entrance to the vagina, and are commonly referred to as genital warts. These are most commonly caused by HPV Types 6 and 11 and have the appearance of raised, flattened small lumps. Over 60% of women with genital warts generally require one or two local treatments to eradicate them.

This involves the application of a chemical substance (either podophyllin or trichloracetic acid) to the warts, which may cause a stinging sensation which can persist for some hours after treatment. The treated area may also be tender for some days afterwards, stinging each time you pass urine. Intercourse may also be uncomfortable and further irritate the recently treated area. Sixty percent of women respond to one or two treatments; 20% will require several treatments; whilst the remaining 20% will have their genital warts spontaneously regress.

The presence of genital warts **DOES NOT** predispose you to the development of **CIN** (dysplasia) of the cervix.

Causes and Prevention

As we have seen, the presence of HPV in a woman's genital tract is not uncommon, with the mode of transmission unclear.

Several medical studies have observed the presence of HPV in the genital tract of virgins and children with no evidence of sexual contact. However, it is thought that HPV can be sexually transmitted from one partner to another and there really is no way of knowing whether your partner has this virus, unless he has visible warts on his penis. Even in the absence of genital warts on your partner's penis, it is still possible that he may have HPV, which can be transmitted to you through sexual intercourse, and can manifest visibly as genital warts or invisibly, and only be detected microscopically on your Pap smear.

The presence of HPV **does not** imply you or your partner is sexually promiscuous — just that you are unlucky to sleep with a partner who does have the virus. Since our sexual relationships involve trust, fears of violation of that trust can often be uppermost in your mind if you do develop genital warts.

Prevention? Now that we live with AIDS in our community, **safe sex** is a must — so make sure your partner wears a condom!

When HPV is identified on a Pap smear, a repeat smear in six months is usually recommended and if HPV changes persist, then investigation with a colposcope is indicated.

I have been in a long-term relationship for many years, but we do not live together.

I developed genital warts six months ago and have HPV changes to the cells of my cervix.

I am scared I will develop cervical cancer now, because my doctor told me this might happen.

My genital warts are everywhere; they just keep appearing all the time. I haven't slept with anyone else and my boyfriend said he hasn't either. It seems strange that after all these years of our relationship I should suddenly develop them.

When I told my boyfriend I had warts, there was a "dead silence" — I didn't hear from him for weeks and he didn't return my calls. We use condoms now and our relationship is strained. Intercourse is uncomfortable because the warts become irritated and it hurts. I feel unclean, ashamed and dirty. I haven't slept with anyone else and now I feel like I have a contagious disease. I feel humiliated and dirty.

I feel so embarrassed when I see my doctor for treatment ... and they keep returning ... and I keep having more treatment.

One Woman's Comments

• *Positive Results*

A positive result will usually reflect the detection of abnormal cells which have been sampled from a CIN or pre-cancerous area of the cervix (see Figures 8, 9, 10).

Since a Pap smear is a screening test only, it cannot <u>make</u> a diagnosis.

The presence of CIN of any degree (1, 2, 3, micro-invasive or invasive cancer) requires referral for investigation. Abnormal cells of the cervix are invisible to the naked eye and therefore need investigation involving the inspection of the cervix with a microscope called a colposcope (see Figures 19 and 20).

• *CIN 1 (Mild Dysplasia)*

If your Pap smear reveals CIN 1 and your doctor recommends a repeat smear in three or six months, ask him why. It is preferable to have a colposcopic examination if any degree of CIN is present and most authorities would suggest this course of action.

• *CIN 2 (Moderate Dysplasia)*

If your smear result reports the presence of CIN 2 or moderate dysplasia, ask for a referral to a gynaecologist to ascertain the degree of abnormality of the cells and to have a colposcopic examination.

- ### *CIN 3 (Severe Dysplasia)*
  (Previously known as Carcinoma Insitu)
  You should be referred immediately to a gynaecologist so that you can have a colposcopic examination and the nature of the abnormality can be diagnosed and treated.

> I am 32 and recently had a Pap smear test which revealed abnormal cells in the canal of the cervix. I was referred to a gynaecologist and had a cone biopsy.
>
> At my check-up a few weeks later, I was told that the cone biopsy confirmed abnormal cells which had been removed.
>
> I am a little puzzled though—because when my girlfriend had an abnormal Pap smear, she had a colposcopic examination done to look at the abnormal cells of the cervix first—before she had a cone biopsy—should I have had this done too?

One Woman's Comments

- ### *Micro-Invasive/Invasive Cancer*
  You should be referred immediately to a gynaecologist for further investigation by colposcopic examination — a gynaecologist-oncologist possesses more expertise in this area than a gynaecologist-obstetrician.

Questions to ask your doctor when a smear is abnormal—

- What is the nature of the abnormality?

- What causes this abnormality?

- Do I need another smear test and when?

- If my Pap smear reveals CIN (dysplasia) or atypical cells, I would like a referral to a gynaecologist for further investigation.

- What other investigations may be performed?

- May I have a copy of my Pap smear result? **(Always ask for a copy of your Pap smear result when abnormal; such a request is reasonable and may be useful in the future.)**

Figure 18—Questions to Ask

• *False Negative Pap Smears*

A false negative Pap smear result is one which mistakenly reports that the presence of CIN or malignant cells of the cervix are not evident, when in fact they are present.

In Australia the official false negative rate for Pap smear results is believed to be 10% and such results can occur for a variety of reasons:

— *An inadequate sample of cells taken*

This can be due to poor technique or inadequate experience of the health professional taking the Pap smear; or the transformation zone may not be sampled adequately, ie the presence of columnar cells and squamous cells and cells of the transformation zone are not present on a smear.

— *Associated conditions*

The presence of inflammation (infection), blood, post-menopausal atrophy of the cells, can all obscure the presence of CIN.

— *Inadequate fixation*

When cells of the cervix are sampled by taking a Pap smear, the cells are placed on a glass slide and sprayed with a fixative to preserve them. Inadequate fixative or artificial drying of the slide may result in a false negative result.

— *Screening by the cytopathologist*

The **experience** of the cytopathologist / pathologist / technician who examines the smear for abnormal cells, is of great importance in observing and reporting **any** abnormal cell change. Quality control within pathology laboratories is of immense importance — some laboratories are recognised for their expertise in this field, whereas others may examine Pap smears infrequently.

The volume of Pap smears examined by each pathologist during a day varies between laboratories. It is generally accepted that human fatigue and error can occur if more than 50 smears are examined by a pathologist in one day. There may be one or two abnormal cells amongst thousands of normal cells present on a Pap smear, so it is therefore vital that good quality control exists within pathology laboratories which examine them.

— *Communication of results*

You should not assume "no news is good news". Since you have a Pap smear test taken in the interest of your health, so should you telephone for the results of your Pap smear test a week after it has been taken. Obtaining the results of your Pap smear test is **your responsibility**.

— *Pap smear results*

Sometimes there may be a failure to report an abnormal Pap smear result when this is indicated, or there may be a failure to investigate and refer you to a gynaecologist when CIN is evident on a Pap smear.

The chance of a having false negative Pap smear result is reduced dramatically by:

- Experienced medical practitioners.

- Reliable cytopathology services.

- Frequent Pap smear tests, ie yearly or two-yearly. The false negative incidence is reduced and eliminated by regular screening.

- Good communication and monitoring of results, ie Pap Smear Registry.

Whilst false negative results are lower in Australia than in other countries, it is unfortunate that false negative results occur at all. Yet, because such results **are** negative, the presence of symptoms has not been fully investigated. In the presence of symptoms, a false negative result may still occur, due to an inadequate smear, pathology error or, unusually, a rapidly developing cervical cancer.

Abnormal symptoms need investigation, irrespective of Pap smear results, ie a negative smear does not cancel abnormal symptoms.

Medical Litigation

In May 1994, in a New South Wales' court, a medical precedent was set in Australia by a young woman, terminally ill with cervical cancer. She was awarded costs against a pathology laboratory who returned an incorrect Pap smear result, and her doctor, who failed to investigate her continuing abnormal symptoms.

Again in May 1994, this time in Victoria, another young woman, now terminally ill with cervical cancer diagnosed during her pregnancy following a false negative Pap smear result, was awarded an out-of-court settlement.

As a result of this recent litigation, which was reported in the media, many women have reacted in one of two ways: women are now presenting to their doctor or nurse for six-monthly Pap smears, whilst others are cancelling their appointments to have their routine Pap smears.

Whilst **no** screening test is perfect, the Pap smear is the only test we have at the moment. It is all too easy for women in the face of this recent successful litigation, to make a decision not to bother with having a Pap smear test, because it is not perfect. Well, nothing in our life is perfect is it? No matter how hard we try for it?

To make a decision not to have a Pap smear test based on this, is nothing short of a cop-out — a poor excuse. No woman particularly **likes** having a Pap smear test, so it is a convenient excuse to use the 10% false negative rate to avoid having regular Pap smears tests.

If, on the other hand, you do have a Pap smear result which indicates the presence of abnormal cells and these are subsequently confirmed by a gynaecologist, you will feel most relieved. If these changes had remained undetected and untreated they could have progressed to cancer.

Do yourself a favour — don't "cop-out" — take responsibility for your health and **always** question when in doubt and seek another opinion, or another even, until you are satisfied.

For those of you who have won or lost, or nearly won or lost the battle or the war with cancer, and who now consider seeking retribution for negligence you perceive to have been occasioned by your treating physician, remember it is a long, hard and expensive battle you are now contemplating. It is a battle fraught with emotion where you will have to re-live your experience over and again in endless repetitive detail; emotional, physical and intimate detail — to strangers — and in front of strangers.

Even if you can establish that your doctor failed in his duty of care, was indeed negligent and that you have suffered damage as a result, you have to find a doctor who is willing to testify to this in a court of law. It is accepted that few doctors or pathologists will testify against fellow practitioners — they have their own reputations and practices to uphold — a life's foundation which can become very precarious if testifying against a fellow practitioner.

Given that you are able to find a doctor to testify on your behalf, you need to be in a financially sound position. Most women who do give serious thought to medical litigation generally abandon such thoughts because of the huge costs involved in such litigation, although some barristers will offer their services on a contingency fee basis.

Assuming you can afford the legal fees and can find a doctor willing to testify on your behalf, the stress of a court case should not be dismissed lightly. If you are cured of your cancer, you may just be grateful that you are still alive and choose not to pursue legal avenues. Similarly, if you have progressive cancer requiring continuing treatment or palliative care — all your energies are taken up with living life to the fullest — now.

If, having chosen not to proceed with a medical negligence case, you still feel angry, why not speak to the doctor concerned and explain how you feel? If you feel so upset that you are unable to do this, some States have a confidential health complaints service, where personnel can advise you and approach the doctor on your behalf. A written complaint to the Australian Medical Association (AMA) in your State may result in investigation of your complaint.

If you do choose to proceed with a medical negligence case, consider whether this will resolve your anger and make you happier. You cannot undo what has been done, nor can you change the circumstances which occurred. Will going to court lead you to accepting your situation more fully? Is your anger at trying to hurt the doctor or pathologist not going to hurt you? Anger stops us from resolving conflict and prevents personal growth.

> Life is too short to be absorbed by anger and bitterness.

I had been on the contraceptive pill for many years and decided to take a break.

Soon after, I developed a watery vaginal discharge, which was constant. I assumed the hormonal function of my ovaries was returning to normal now that I was not on the pill.

I had two Pap smears in eleven months — both were negative.

The watery discharge was constant and obvious, with an unpleasant odour, and I wore a sanitary pad at times.

Since my Pap smear results were normal I was not in the least concerned. I did not bother to tell my doctor — I had no irregular spotting or bleeding.

To cut a long story short, it was eventually discovered that I had an unusually rapid growing invasive cancer of the cervix.

I subsequently had the two smears re-assessed by two different pathologists. The last one, when rechecked, showed a frank invasive carcinoma of the squamous cells and columnar cells of the transformation zone.

I still do not know how they could have made such a mistake; I guess I never will.

One Woman's Comments

PART III

Diagnostic Investigations

Since we know that a Pap smear test is a screening test only, in the event that the presence of CIN of any degree is identified or your Pap smear returns a negative result, yet abnormal symptoms continue, it is accepted medical practice that you will be referred to a gynaecologist, whose area of expertise is CIN or dysplasia of the cervix, and who will further investigate the nature and severity of the abnormal cervical cells reported. Further investigation should involve one or more of the following procedures:

- A colposcopic examination.

- A punch biopsy of abnormal cells.

- A cone biopsy of abnormal cells (see page 71).

Colposcopic Examination

A Colposcopic (colpo=vagina, scope=look) examination is the inspection of the cervix through a binocular-microscope called a colposcope. It is used to identify the location, size and area of the abnormality of the cervix, including the transformation zone, following an abnormal Pap smear result or abnormal symptons. The colposcope magnifies the cervix eight to thirty times for easy identification of abnormal cells. This procedure is performed in the Outpatients' Department of your hospital, or in a gynaecologist's surgery, takes approximately 15 minutes and is uncomfortable, but not painful. You are awake and no anaesthetic is required.

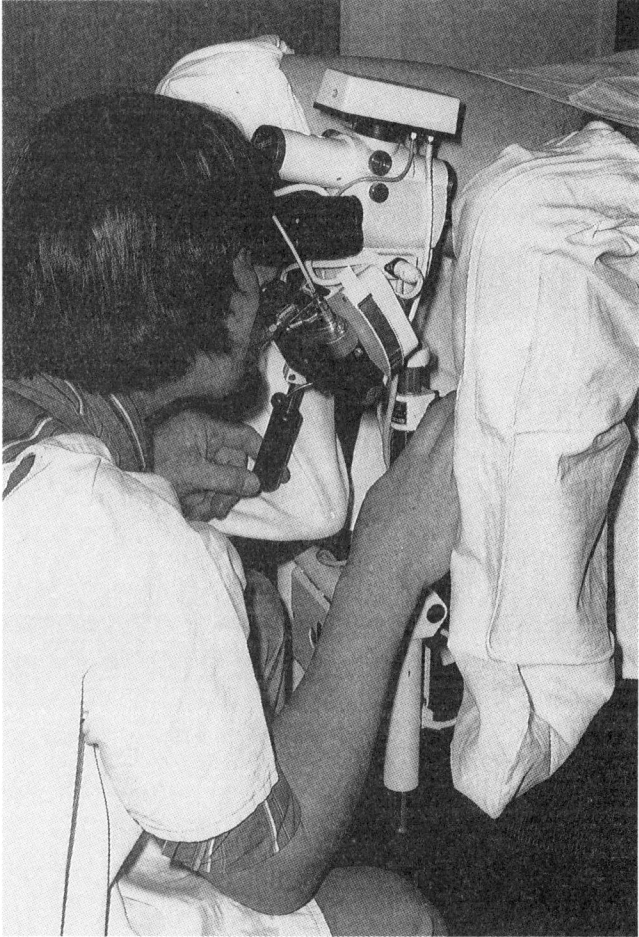

Figure 19—Colposcopic Examination
Photograph courtesy of Professor R Planner, University of Melbourne, Department of Gynaecology-Oncology, Mercy Hospital for Women

Colposcopic Examination Procedure

This involves undressing from the waist down and lying on an examination table; or sitting in a chair designed for colposcopic examination. Your legs are parted and your feet will rest on foot rests. Some women may feel embarrassed and somewhat exposed during this examination.

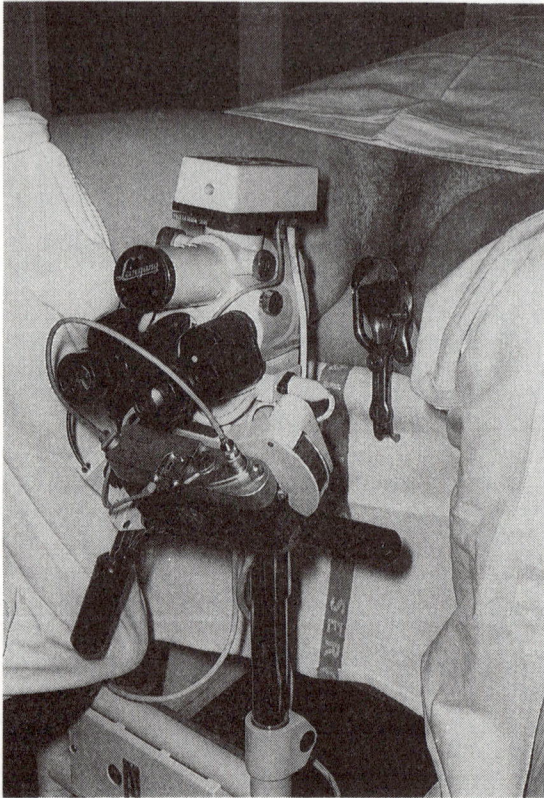

Figure 20—Colposcopic Examination—view 2

A speculum has been inserted to separate the walls of the vagina. Photograph courtesy of Professor R Planner, University of Melbourne, Department of Gynaecology-Oncology, Mercy Hospital for Women

A speculum is then inserted into your vagina to separate the walls of the vagina and the colposcope is positioned between your legs; the doctor then looks through the binocular-microscope which magnifies your cervix to identify any abnormal areas. Some doctors will have a closed-circuit television and a large screen, so that you can also watch and observe what is going on. Many women find it interesting to look at their cervix on the television screen, and this gives the doctor the opportunity to explain to you what is being seen and done during the procedure.

The doctor will generally take a Pap smear at this point, and then swab the cervix with a saline solution (this may cause a brief stinging sensation) to remove mucus produced by the cervix. This gives a clear view of the cervix so the colour and general appearance can be observed. The cervix is then swabbed with acetic acid (vinegar solution) which, when applied to any abnormal cells on the cervix, shows up as white. Iodine may also be applied to the cervix, to help visualise any abnormal areas.

Punch Biopsy

If the colposcopic examination reveals any abnormal areas of the cervix, a punch biopsy will be taken. A punch biopsy involves taking very tiny samples (biopsy) of any abnormal area observed during the colposcopic examination. It may be painless, or at most mildly uncomfortable and some women have likened it to period pain. Colposcopic examinations and punch biopsies are also totally safe procedures during pregnancy, not harming your cervix or your baby.

> **Diagnosis of CIN can <u>only</u> be established by a punch biopsy, after which appropriate treatment can be planned.**

I was referred to a dysplasia clinic at a women's hospital in the city because my Pap smear result was abnormal. My doctor told me I would need a colposcopic examination to ascertain **why** my Pap smear result was abnormal.

I was scared I had cancer and I thought a colposcopic examination was an operation. I wish my doctor had given me a leaflet or something that explained what might happen. I had no idea and assumed the worst.

The doctor at the dysplasia clinic was great and explained what would happen. I sat in a special chair and with a binocular microscope called a colposcope, the doctor looked at my cervix. This was transmitted to a television set and I was able to see my own cervix, whilst the doctor explained everything. I found it all very interesting, and despite an abnormal Pap smear, the doctor was able to see that there were no abnormal cells at all!!

One Woman's Comments

After the colposcopic examination is completed you can dress and your doctor will explain to you what has been found. Many women will often take their partner or friend along for reassurance; two people listening to the doctor can make it easier to comprehend and remember than one. Most of the time invasive cancer can be ruled out or confirmed during colposcopic examination, as often, if present, it can be immediately identified.

After Colposcopic Examination
You may experience intermittent mild cramp (like period pain) for a day or so; you may experience slight spotting or a dark discharge for a day or two; and this is all quite normal. To allow healing of the biopsy areas you should also avoid intercourse for a week after punch biopsy, as well as the use of tampons, should your period occur.

Final analysis of your punch biopsy results should be available within a week, and the results will indicate what, if any, treatment is required for the abnormality of the cells of the cervix. No treatment should be planned until the colposcopic examination and biopsy results are known. The technique of a general anaesthetic, colposcopic examination, biopsy and treatment, **all at the same time**, is not to be recommended as it may lead to inappropriate treatment. Another appointment will be made for you to receive and discuss your results and for any treatment required.

> **You should contact your doctor if, following a punch biopsy you continue to bleed (not your period) or if you develop an offensive discharge, feel unwell and/or have a high temperature.**

Cone Biopsy

A cone biopsy involves the removal of a cone-shaped piece of tissue from the cervix and is performed for diagnostic purposes; it often **simultaneously removes** CIN or abnormal cells.

Please refer to page 71 for further details of this procedure.

Questions to ask your doctor—
It may be helpful if you have a prepared list of questions to ask your doctor after your colposcopic examination, because if you are nervous, you may forget to ask any questions you may have thought about prior to or during the examination.

● What does the colposcopic examination reveal?

● Is the abnormality likely to be cancer?

● When will the results of the punch biopsy be available?

● What physical after-effects can I expect following the punch biopsy?

● What degree or level of CIN or dysplasia does it appear that I have?

● Will I need treatment? What treatment?

● Can CIN or dysplasia recur after treatment?

● Is treatment totally successful?

● Is there anything I can do to prevent the recurrence of dysplasia?

● After treatment of the dysplasia, do I need further colposcopic examinations?

● How often should I have Pap smears after treatment of the dysplasia?

● If I have to wait two or three months for treatment of CIN, can it progress to cancer?

● If the wart virus is present, does this need to be treated?

● If the wart virus does not need treatment, how often should I have Pap smears?

● Does the wart virus pre-dispose me to developing CIN?

Figure 21—Questions to Ask

Abnormal Pap Smears During Pregnancy

Diagnosis will generally follow a routine Pap smear test performed at the time of physical examination when confirmation of your pregnancy occurs. Pap smear tests during pregnancy are safe and most abnormal smears can be safely left for treatment until after the baby is born.

If CIN is identified, pregnancy will not affect its progress; however, a referral for a colposcopic examination would generally be indicated. Minor areas of cervical cell abnormality at colposcopic examination during pregnancy can be observed and safely left untreated until after the birth.

In women where micro-invasive or invasive cancer is suspected during their colposcopic examination, a punch biopsy will be taken to confirm this diagnosis and the appropriate treatment planned. A punch biopsy will not harm you or your baby during pregnancy — you are **not** at risk of miscarriage from a punch biopsy of the cervix.

A cone biopsy is generally **not** performed during pregnancy as the transformation zone is located on the ectocervix and is easily identified during colposcopic examination.

I had a Pap smear when my pregnancy was confirmed and this was normal. However, at my post-natal check-up, another Pap smear was taken which revealed an abnormal result. My gynaecologist told me this was nothing to worry about and that I should have a repeat smear in three months time, which I did; this was also abnormal.

I have since had three further abnormal Pap smear results and my gynaecologist performed a colposcopic examination after the fifth abnormal Pap smear result. I was admitted to hospital two days later for a cone biopsy, where part of my cervix was removed because it was almost cancer.

I still don't quite understand much about this. My gynaecologist said it is nothing to worry about, but I do worry because I still don't understand completely.

One Woman's Comments

Treatment of CIN

Final analysis of your punch biopsy results should be available within a week and the results will indicate what, if any, treatment is required for the abnormality found.

There are several treatments available to successfully treat and eradicate CIN. These are:

- Laser
- Diathermy
- Cryo-surgery or cryo-cautery
- Cone biopsy.

Laser

The use of laser beams to destroy CIN (abnormal cells) has largely replaced the more conventional treatments of diathermy and cryo-surgery. The use of the laser is restricted to doctors who are very skilled in its use. The advantages of laser treatment include its precision. Treatment takes a short time and healing of the cervix occurs quickly. Most major women's hospitals now have laser treatment available to women.

What happens during treatment?

This treatment is usually performed in the Outpatient's Department of a hospital and may involve either the administration of a general anaesthetic or a local anaesthetic. A colposcopic examination is performed and during this, the use of the laser eradicates the abnormal cells identified on visual inspection, which have been confirmed by a punch biopsy.

Following laser treatment, you can expect a watery or dark vaginal discharge for a few days or a week following this treatment. You may experience mild period-type discomfort for a day or so and you may like to take the following day off work. Following laser treatment you should not have sexual intercourse for three weeks to allow healing of the cervix, and if your menstrual period occurs, you should not use tampons for three weeks .

You will be reviewed by the doctor for a Pap smear test at three, six and twelve months following laser treatment and a repeat colposcopic examination is generally performed six months after laser treatment. You should have yearly Pap smears tests after treatment for CIN.

Diathermy

The use of diathermy to destroy CIN is achieved by using a fine electric current. A more recent method gaining in popularity, is a loop excision which removes strips of the abnormal cells of the cervix with a fine wire, through which an electro surgical current is passed.

What happens during treatment?

This treatment is performed in the Outpatient's Department of a hospital and involves the administration of a general anaesthetic. The abnormal area is again visualised, which has been confirmed by a punch biopsy.

Following diathermy you can expect a dark vaginal discharge and perhaps a grey-greenish discharge which has a sweet odour, for up to six weeks. You may experience mild period-type discomfort for a day or so and you might like to take the following day off work.

Following treatment you should not have sexual intercourse for three weeks to allow healing of the cervix and you should not use tampons for three weeks if your menstrual period occurs.

Your follow up care includes a Pap smear at three, six and twelve months following a diathermy of the cervix and a repeat coloscopic examination is generally performed six months after this treatment. However, follow-up care can vary with each doctor, and depending upon the grade of CIN treated, so you should discuss this with your doctor. You should have at least yearly Pap smears tests after treatment for CIN.

Cryo-surgery (Cryo-cautery)

In this method, abnormal cells of the cervix are destroyed by a freezing technique, using carbon dioxide or nitrous oxide. This method of treatment is used less commonly since the advent of laser surgery.

What happens during treatment?

As with laser and diathermy, cryo-surgery is usually performed in the Outpatient's Department of a hospital and generally involves the administration of either a general or local anaesthetic. The area to be treated is identified through a colposcopic examination following a previous punch biopsy to confirm the presence of CIN.

Following this treatment you can expect a watery or dark vaginal discharge for up to a week and you may experience mild period-type discomfort for a day or so.

You should not have sexual intercourse for three weeks following treatment, to allow healing of your cervix and you should avoid the use of tampons for three weeks if your period occurs.

Cone Biopsy

A cone biopsy involves the removal of a cone-shaped piece of tissue from the cervix, and this is usually performed under a general anaesthetic, either surgically or by laser.

A cone biopsy is a diagnostic evaluation of:

● The columnar cells in the endocervical canal.

● The transformation zone (squamous and columnar cells) when located in the endocervical canal.

In what circumstances is a cone biopsy performed?
A cone biopsy is performed:

● When a Pap smear reports CIN of the columnar cells situated in the endocervical canal and a colposcopic examination may not be able to fully visualise the entire abnormal area.

● If micro-invasive cancer of the cervix is suspected during colposcopic examination.

● If a Pap smear test reports CIN or micro-invasive cancer of the cervix, yet a colposcopic examination reveals no abnormality of the cells, a cone biopsy is required for definitive diagnosis.

● If a punch biopsy reveals micro-invasive cancer of the cervix.

During the course of a cone biopsy your doctor will often be able to diagnose and **simultaneously remove** CIN/abnormal cells or micro-invasive cancer.

If invasive cancer is suspected, a cone biopsy will enable your doctor to evaluate the depth and extent of early invasive cancer.

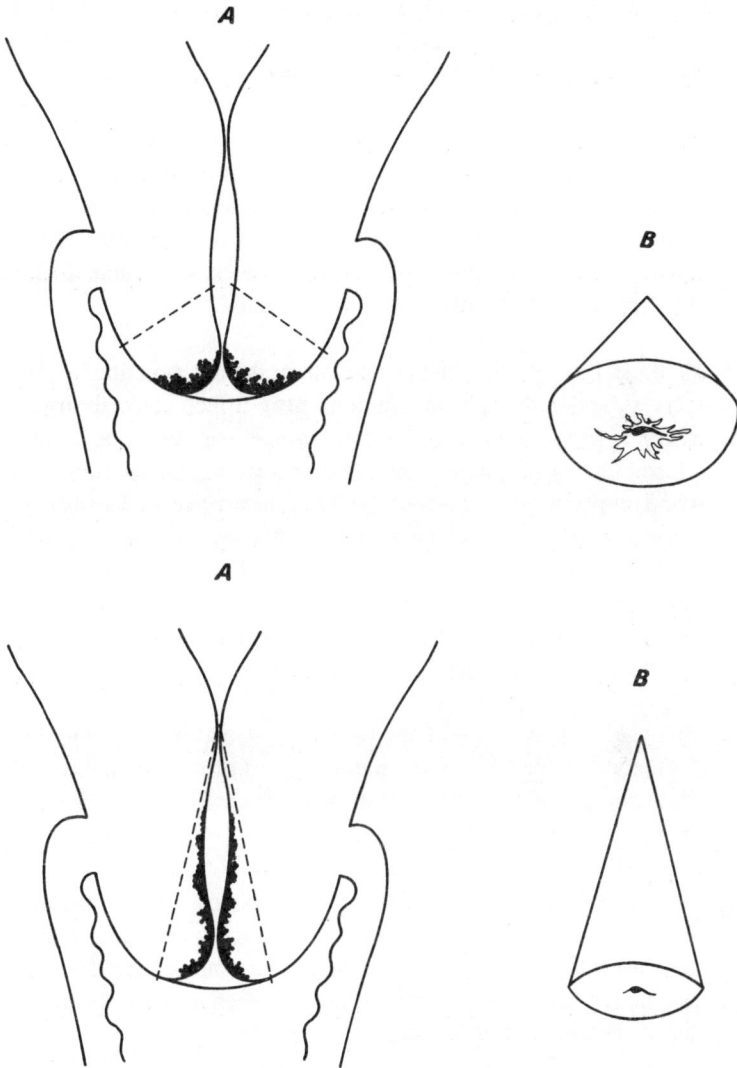

Figure 22—Cone Biopsy

A: This involves the removal of a cone-shaped segment of tissue from the cervix.

B: Cone-shaped segment of tissue taken from the cervix.

Since a cone biopsy is performed under a general anaesthetic it normally involves an overnight stay in hospital. From a medical perspective it is a minor diagnostic and/or treatment procedure, but it may have possible side effects:

- Since a cone-shaped piece of tissue is removed from the cervix, it may affect the mucus-producing function of the columnar cells in the endocervix. Women who rely on the mucus method of contraception will need to check with their doctor that this form of contraception is still reliable.

- A cone biopsy can change the strength and function of the cervix, and although uncommon, **may** affect your ability to carry a pregnancy to full term. Since the cervix is tightly closed during pregnancy, removal of a wedge of the cervix by cone biopsy might predispose you to miscarriage — because the cervix is unable to close tightly and keep the foetus in the uterus. Women who become pregnant following a cone biopsy, may have a stitch placed in the cervix at 14-16 weeks of pregnancy to prevent miscarriage; the stitch is removed at 38-40 weeks of pregnancy.

- Stenosis or narrowing of the tissue of the cervix caused by the formation of scar tissue can manifest itself as reduced menstrual flow and an increase in period pain. Stenosis of the cervix is more common in older women.

- You may be at a greater risk of developing a pelvic infection because the protective function of the cervix is absent. Vaginal infections, if not treated promptly, can become pelvic infections which can lead to infertility caused by infection of the fallopian tubes; however, this is rare.

> Having a cone biopsy does not necessarily mean any of these problems will occur, they are included to make you aware of what could happen.

Before you have a cone biopsy you should discuss its pros and cons at length with your doctor. The advantages of cone biopsy, as a means of accurate diagnosis and effective treatment of abnormalities of the cervix, will mostly outweigh the potential disadvantages.

> If the doctor performing your colposcopic examination suggests a cone biopsy, it may be in your best interests to ask for a referral to a gynaecologist-oncologist — particularly if **micro-invasive** cancer is suspected.

Whilst a gynaecologist, especially one who specialises in colposcopic examinations and cervical CIN/dysplasia, is well-qualified and experienced in performing cone biopsies, in the event that it confirms you have micro-invasive or invasive cancer, the expertise of a gynaecologist-oncologist, who specialises in all aspects of reproductive cancer, may be regarded as treatment *par excellence*.

> Cone biopsy, as treatment for micro-invasive cancer, is dependent upon good planning based on colposcopic examinations and **expert** evaluation of the "cone" by a skilled pathologist. It is also essential that all abnormal tissue and a margin of normal tissue of the cervix is removed to ensure a complete cure. A gynaecologist-oncologist, working closely with a skilled pathologist, would ensure optimum treatment.

If I seem to be emphasising the point, it is because I have spoken with some women on whom cone biopsy was performed "successfully" by a gynaecologist (without oncology expertise), and who later developed metastatic cancer because the cancer was not totally removed at cone biopsy. It only takes one cancer cell in normal tissue for this to occur, hence the removal of a margin of normal tissue at cone biopsy. If the margins are not clear, more radical surgery may be needed.

If your gynaecologist suspects invasive cancer, you should be made aware of this and you may have to wait two to three weeks until you can be seen by a gynaecologist-oncologist. If you do have cancer it does not mean that it is growing wildly out of control during this time. Whilst you will be very frightened and fearful and willing to have a cone biopsy as soon as possible, as recommended by your gynaecologist, do seek a referral to a gynaecologist-oncologist — it may be in your best interest.

Cone Biopsy Treatment

You are generally admitted to hospital the morning of the cone biopsy, will stay overnight and be discharged the following day. It is a short procedure and requires a general anaesthetic, although in some overseas countries it is performed under a local anaesthetic. You may have dissolvable stitches in the cervix and you can expect some minor vaginal blood loss for a week or so. You may experience moderate cramp (like period pain) and/or backache, which can be controlled by a narcotic injection — one is usually sufficient; and you may need to take simple pain killers four-hourly as needed over the next few days.

Questions to ask your doctor—

● Why is it absolutely essential to have a cone biopsy?

● What are the possible physical side effects of this treatment?

● Do you suspect that I have micro-invasive cancer of the cervix?

● In the event that a cone biopsy reveals invasive cancer or micro-invasive cancer—

   — What will happen?

   — Who will treat me?

      ● A gynaecologist who specialises in CIN/dysplasia?

      ● A gynaecologist-oncologist?

● Are you a gynaecologist-oncologist?

● If you are not, would you please give me copies of the results of my Pap smear test/s, colposcopic examination and my punch biopsy, and a referral letter to a gynaecologist-oncologist for a second opinion.

                    or

Make an appointment with your local doctor and ask for a referral to a gynaecologist-oncologist. Your local doctor will then obtain copies of your previous reports.

Figure 23—Questions to Ask

Emotions

Most women feel very anxious as they await the results of their cone biopsy. Women in this situation, where their doctor suspects micro-invasive cancer, and whose cone biopsy was performed for this purpose, should have been made aware of the possibility of this prior to surgery. You will also hope that cone biopsy will be sufficient treatment, particularly if you do not have children. Anxiety, fear and shock at the possibility of cancer can be quite overwhelming at this time, as you wait for the results of your cone biopsy.

Results of Cone Biopsy

Results of your cone biopsy will usually be available within seven days. The doctor's receptionist will generally ring you to make an appointment to discuss results when they are available. Most of the time a cone biopsy, taken for diagnostic purposes, is sufficient treatment in itself for micro-invasive cancer up to 3mm in depth from the basement membrane. Follow-up will require three- to six-monthly colposcopic examinations for a year; then six-monthly Pap smear tests.

Care at home
You will usually need to—

- Take things quietly for a week following cone biopsy and if you work, it is advisable to take the week off.

- Refrain from performing heavy housework tasks, eg lifting wet washing, moving heavy furniture, etc.

- For the next six weeks, refrain from using tampons when you have your period, to allow healing of the cervix.

- Prevent ascending infection by avoiding swimming and lying in the bath.

- Allow complete healing of the cervix by avoiding sexual intercourse until cleared by your doctor (usually six weeks).

Figure 24—Care at Home

If invasive cancer is diagnosed, more radical treatment will be required. Many gynaecologists who perform cone biopsies will automatically refer you to a gynaecologist-oncologist if invasive cancer is apparent. However, some will not.

Correct treatment of invasive cervical cancer involves the team work of a histopathologist and two gynaecologist-oncologists in consultation together, so that correct "staging" of your cancer occurs, allowing optimum treatment of your condition.

Follow-up care after treatment for CIN

Following treatment for CIN/abnormal cells of the cervix and when the tissues have healed, normal squamous cells with redevelop. In order to ensure that CIN has been eradicated, you will require follow-up appointments with your doctor. This includes having Pap smear tests at three-, six- and twelve-monthly intervals, as well as another colposcopic examination at approximately six months.

Follow-up care may vary with each doctor and depending on the grade of CIN treated, so you should discuss this together. Any woman diagnosed and treated for CIN should have annual Pap smears for the rest of her life.

The majority of women will require only one treatment for CIN, depending on the type of treatment used and the grade of CIN present. In some women, however, despite successful treatment, CIN may recur, necessitating further treatment. It is therefore **most important** to follow your doctor's recommendation of attending for repeat Pap smear tests and colposcopic examinations.

My doctor told me I had cervical intra-epithelial neoplasia (CIN), Stage 3, four years ago, which was successfully treated with laser under a general anaesthetic.

I have always assumed that this meant I had a Stage 3 cancer, particularly since I bled very heavily after the punch biopsy, which required hospitalisation and minor surgery.

At each follow-up appointment during the last four years, I have been petrified that more cancer will be found and I would need a hysterectomy — I am single and have no children.

I've just read your book on cervical cancer and CIN and after four years of incredible worry I finally understand and realise that I did **not** have cancer after all. "Cervical intra-epithelial neoplasia" is the medical term for abnormal cells of the cervix — **not** cancer cells!

Whilst I am now feeling relief **four years later** — I do wish I had asked more questions at the time and not **assumed** the worst!

One Woman's Comments

PART IV

Emotions Felt
When CIN is Diagnosed

For many women, an abnormal Pap smear result for the first time, can raise many fears, concerns and anxieties — which are often unspoken.

An abnormal Pap smear result for most women, is totally unexpected; for years you may have had regular or intermittent Pap smear tests in the interests of your health and well-being and most often with little, if any thought, that it might one day be positive. Of course, when this does occur, often you can be thrown into absolute emotional turmoil, feel very vulnerable and powerless or even have feelings of a loss of control over your body.

You may wonder:

• How on earth could I have an abnormal Pap smear?

• What caused it?

• What exactly is an abnormal Pap smear?

As we have seen in previous chapters, an abnormal Pap smear may reflect an inconclusive result or infection, inflammation, post-menopausal or post-partum atrophy, in which case the cause can be treated simply and effectively.

In women whose abnormal Pap smear result indicates the presence of CIN (dysplasia), it can raise other fears. For example, you may wonder why abnormal cells have developed in **your** cervix, or you may even wonder if you have done "something" to cause this.

You may worry about referrals to another doctor and investigate medical procedures such as a colposcopic examination, punch biopsy or cone biopsy — all of which you have possibly never heard of before and all of which may sound terribly frightening and very serious. You may even have very strong fears that cancer will be found.

The issues of an abnormal Pap smear result are often personal to you alone, and yet often are the same feelings other women in this situation also have. Some issues in particular may assume extreme importance and be a source of great worry and anxiety to you, whilst other women may have different individual issues or concerns. Yet others will give it little thought, with few, if any, concerns at all.

The emotions and feelings you have at this time are very normal and to help you regain some sense of equilibrium and normality, I will, in the next few pages, explore some of the issues which may be of concern to you, so that together, we can make some sense of it, and you can have some peace of mind.

Abnormal Cells Do <u>Not</u> Mean Cancer

As we have already seen in previous chapters, a Pap smear test is a **screening test** only — it is **not** a definitive diagnosis of the presence of CIN/abnormal cells — this can only be made following a visual examination of the cervix through a colposcope and a biopsy of any abnormal cells which become apparent when acetic acid or an iodine solution is applied to the cervix.

Of the millions of cells observed by the cytopathologist who examines your Pap smear through a microscope, there may be only three or four abnormal cells. Scientifically it is a fact that our bodies produce abnormal cells at different times in our lives, which our immune system destroys.

Similarly, if a Pap smear test does reveal abnormal cells, often they can spontaneously revert to normal and will not be apparent during a colposcopic examination. It is also a valid point to note that the development of CIN 1 of the squamous cells for example, and their possible progression to CIN 3 if untreated, does **not** occur overnight — it can take many months or even two years or so to develop. Therefore, regular **screening** by having Pap smear tests, reduces the possibility that a cancer of the cervix has developed. Whilst it can be difficult not to worry that your abnormal Pap smear result may reveal cancer, it is pertinent to remember that over 90% of abnormal cells found on Pap smears and colposcopic examinations are **not cancer**.

Doctor — Patient Relationship

Women often report a sense of shock and disbelief when told their Pap smear has abnormalities. Since you are unprepared for this, you often do not know what questions to ask; nor are you able to have an informed discussion on its meaning, so you are largely guided by what your doctor tells you. Many doctors will explain the nature of the abnormality with diagrams, and recommend the best course of action depending upon your result.

As we already know it is accepted medical practice based on expert opinion, that a referral to a doctor or gynaecologist who specialises in colposcopic examinations, or a referral to a "dysplasia clinic" at a women's hospital, is regarded as standard medical procedure when CIN is identified on a Pap smear test. This however, does not always occur.

I recall a discussion I had recently with a young lady in her early twenties who asked my advice because she had an abnormal Pap smear result which indicated Grade 3 dysplasia and she did not understand what this meant.

It transpired that six months previously she had had an abnormal result and the smear test was repeated six weeks later — again, an abnormal result. Another Pap smear was taken six weeks later — again, an abnormal result.

An appointment was made for another Pap smear in three months time and she was informed by her doctor that if this was still abnormal, she would probably need a cone biopsy.

She was very concerned at her recurrent abnormal smear results and at the thought of an operation, with very real doubts and fears of the management of her smears.

She also felt unable to have an informed discussion with her GP because she had no understanding of the nature of the abnormality and was frightened; nor did she feel able to ask for a referral to another practitioner.

Sometimes a doctor, whether he believes a condition does not warrant specialist treatment or whether he believes he has the expertise to observe repeated abnormal results which indicate the presence of CIN (dysplasia), neither recommends you see a gynaecologist for investigation of your Pap smear abnormality, nor willingly accepts your suggestion of seeing one.

You may also be in a highly emotive state and perhaps this doctor has been caring for you and your family for many years, or has been a supportive rock to you in the past. You may then hesitate to insist on a referral to a gynaecologist, perhaps feeling you may lose your doctor's support or services. Well ... you may.

Remember though, you have Pap smears taken in the interests of your health and well-being; a preventative health measure; a responsibility you take seriously. It is therefore reasonable to expect your practitioner to respect that responsibility by referring you to the appropriate doctor who has the skills and expertise in colposcopic examinations, when your Pap smear reveals CIN (dysplasia), or if you have abnormal symptoms and a negative Pap smear test result.

On page 51 you will find a list of questions which you may like to ask your doctor, adding others which you think of.

Should a referral not be forthcoming from your doctor when:

● the presence of CIN of any degree (1, 2, 3, micro-invasive or invasive cancer) is identified on your Pap smear; or

● if you have abnormal symptoms (see page 35), irrespective of Pap smear results (a negative Pap smear does not cancel abnormal symptoms),

do seek a second opinion from:

● A doctor at a Well Women's Clinic.

● A Dysplasia Clinic at a Women's Hospital (listed at the back of this book).

● Another GP — and ask him for a referral to a gynaecologist.

Body-image

Women often have little understanding of their reproductive and genital anatomy, including the exact location of their cervix and the nature of CIN or dysplasia of their cervix.

Since you are unable to visualise the abnormal cells of your cervix, this can often cause confusion, misunderstanding and misconception of what abnormal cells look like or indeed their physical effect. You may therefore visualise CIN/abnormal cells growing in clumps which in turn form lumps on your cervix; or even that these cells are somehow "sinister" with the ability to grow and "change" or "deform" your cervix inside your body.

This is of course not true, because basically CIN can be likened to a sun spot on the back of your hand. A sun spot is a **superficial layer** of abnormal cells which you **can** see clearly if it is present on the back of your hand, arms or face. You will mostly not be concerned at its presence for you can observe it for any change in size or colour and seek medical advice when you are concerned. In other words, you feel you have some control because you can readily observe any changes.

However, you cannot see abnormal cells on your cervix, or indeed observe any change, and you have no control. This can therefore raise many different fears causing confusion, misunderstanding and worry. Many doctors who perform colposcopic examinations now have closed circuit television so that you can also see what your doctor is observing, thus giving you the opportunity of actually seeing the abnormal cells of your cervix, if any are present.

Medical advances such as this can often reduce the fear, misunderstanding and worry of the nature of abnormal cells of the cervix, because they enable you to see what abnormal cells actually look like. Nevertheless, for many women an abnormal Pap smear result, followed by investigative medical procedures such as a colposcopic examination with possible biopsy, and the possible diagnosis of CIN and treatment of this, can affect the way you feel about your body-image, self-image and sexuality.

To help you understand why and how this may result, with the permission of Ellen Shipes RN of Vanderbilt University, USA, I have adapted her written understanding of body-image and applied this to the many feelings that you may have during the time you are being investigated and/or treated for CIN. Some of this you may identify with, or you may not, and this is okay because we are all individuals with different feelings, fears and worries during investigation of an abnormal Pap smear result and its treatment.

Body-image is the personal mental picture we have of ourself, and that which we use to identify as being different from others. Our body-image is also intimately associated with our self-esteem, ie our self-esteem is, in part, our feelings about our body and its functions, our relationship and interaction with others and our personal identification, which is shaped by our social, cultural and spiritual beliefs.

If one area of our self-esteem is disrupted, eg how our body functions (the development of abnormal cells within the cervix), it can pose a threat to how we see ourselves — our body-image. Our body-image is always present and constantly changing — from birth throughout life, as we change and mature. During this time changes in our body such as aging occur and such gradual change allows time for our mental image to adjust to our mirror image, so that we maintain self-perception.

As a woman, your reproductive and genital organs have personal value to you in several ways and are part of your body-image.

These organs often represent femininity and your female identity which is symbolic of being a woman through monthly menstruation and your ability to conceive a child where it is nurtured in your uterus before the birth of a new life. Your sexuality is also intimately associated with your femininity and reproductive ability.

However, when abnormal changes to the cells of your cervix occur (CIN), which you cannot see or even visualise and which require treatment, this can result in a different or even distorted image of your body. Feelings of an altered body (image) can result from the perceived threat or the perceived harm you may feel that CIN and its treatment may cause.

Therefore, your personal perception of changes you fear may occur to your cervix, can impact on your female identity, sexuality and body-image. For example, you may feel a loss of control of your body because abnormal cells are developing in your cervix — "How could abnormal cells develop **there**?" — in a part of your body that is personal to you alone and associated with your female identity. You may also have feelings of shame or embarrassment that **this** could happen to you or even guilt feelings, wondering if you have done "something" to cause the development of abnormal cells of the cervix.

You may even feel a sense of shame, unclean and dirty, and feel that your body is a failure and has let you down by the development of abnormal cells in the cherished reproductive area which is part of your female identity.

If you have feelings such as this, and feel that your body is now somehow "different" (changed body-image), it can also impact on your sexual relationship.

Enjoying the emotional and physical release of sex is of primary importance to the balance and well-being of most people. The very intimacy of sex also promotes and enhances sharing, warmth, tenderness, affection, passion and communication, as well as giving us physical release and the ability to be beautiful for the moment. Changes to how you perceive your body (image) at this time can therefore result in a reduced sexual drive or libido, which is your desire or urge for sex.

Your sexual drive is influenced by many factors. If you are emotionally happy, physically healthy and enjoy a good relationship with your partner, you will have sexual desire. However, this will be altered if you are emotionally and/or physically stressed or fatigued, which can often occur during diagnosis and following treatment of CIN. If is therefore not uncommon for women diagnosed with CIN prior to and following treatment, to experience a low sex drive. This can result in loss of spontaneity, reduction in orgasms or even changes to the amount of lubrication produced during sexual arousal, and general lack of interest.

For some of you there are also other fears that can impact on your sexual relationship during this time. You may feel sexually incomplete or even that your body is somehow inadequate, not quite right any more, because you have developed CIN/abnormal cells requiring treatment. Whilst such feelings are quite normal and experienced by many women in this situation, it can occur particularly in women who undergo a cone biopsy for CIN 3 or micro-invasive cancer of the cervix.

It is also not uncommon for temporary changes to occur in your sexual relationship with your partner due to the "cause" of the abnormal cells, ie sexual intercourse. As we already know from extensive medical studies, abnormal cells of the cervix occur in women who have been sexually active. It is also known that cervical cancer occurs rarely in women who have not had sexual intercourse.

Whilst the relationship between squamous cell carcinoma of the cervix and the number of partners a woman has had is well documented in medical literature, it does not apply to many. Many women with abnormal cells of the cervix or cervical cancer have had one partner only and their partner has had only one partner.

Women will sometimes fear health professionals/friends/ partner will be judgemental assuming they have been sexually promiscuous, when in fact they have not. Similarly, in some relationships, partners may "blame" each other for non-existent previous sexual behaviour or indeed be concerned that abnormal cells may develop again through sexual intercourse. You may also fear partner rejection because you feel your body is different. Rest assured that you are still attractive to your partner and the development of abnormal cells and its treatment does **not** reduce your desirability to your partner.

You are **not** contagious, you will not **"catch"** abnormal cells or cervical cancer, by having intercourse.

To enjoy the continuity of your sexual relationship with your partner at this time, communication of your fears and feelings is essential and/or you may like to discuss this with your doctor for added support.

Your feelings towards your body can be many and varied during investigation and treatment of abnormal cells/CIN of the cervix. It is often helpful to know that your feelings are **very normal** and by talking with your partner, close friends, mother or sister and your doctor/nurse, can help enormously. Clear understanding of your condition will often reduce your fears and worries, so that you can regain your equilibrium in what for many is a confusing and upsetting time.

Coping with Fear

Following a colposcopic examination and punch biopsy, which confirms the presence of CIN requiring treatment, you will need close follow-up by your gynaecologist. Your doctor will often repeat smears three-monthly and/or perform further colposcopic examinations at different times, depending upon the grade of CIN of your cervix.

You may find in the interim that you will tend to worry that abnormal cells will recur and if they do, what type of treatment will be required.

If you feel this way, it is worthwhile thinking about how realistic your fears are in relation to your CIN and its treatment.

Clear understanding of your condition and treatment, as well as effective communication with your doctor, will assist in dispelling your fears. If at any time you feel you would like further discussion with your doctor on the presence of CIN and your treatment and are unsure or unconfident in talking about such issues—which are important to you—why not take this book to refer to? Regular attendance for follow-up appointments for Pap smear tests and/or colposcopic examinations, is also important. Some women may be so fearful that they fail to attend regular appointments and in doing so are jeopardising their health.

Many doctors will now give you a copy of your negative Pap smear report automatically, and as time passes with continued negative smear results, your fears will gradually abate to an emotionally manageable level.

If you find a major part of your time is consumed by fear, anxiety, depression or worrying to the exclusion of all else, you will have a less than satisfactory quality of life. It may be worthwhile for you to redirect your energies into positive actions which will interest and benefit you, thereby reducing the time spent worrying and thus reducing your stress levels.

Going for walks, playing sport, listening to relaxation tapes and enjoying relaxation time, may also help manage your fears.

I was diagnosed with CIN following a colposcopic examination and punch biopsy three years ago and successfully treated by laser.

However, since this experience, I have always remained fearful when my 12-monthly Pap smear is due. I dread them! I suppose I am ever fearful that an abnormality will be found again.

One Woman's Comments

PART V

Diagnosis of Cervical Cancer

This chapter is written for women who find themselves in the position where their doctor suspects there is a strong possibility that they have cervical cancer.

In this situation you will generally be made aware that a severe abnormality of the cells of the cervix has been observed during a colposcopic examination. However, as we know, a definite diagnosis can **only** be made through a punch biopsy of those abnormal cells identified during the colposcopic examination.

Often a cone biopsy will follow, to ascertain the depth and extent of the abnormality existing.

DO NOT PANIC!

A cone biopsy will often **simultaneously** diagnose and **remove** CIN/micro-invasive cancer up to a depth of 3mm beyond the basement membrane (see page 72).

If invasive cancer is suspected, a cone biopsy will enable your doctor to evaluate the depth and extent of early invasive cancer of the cervix.

The period of waiting for punch biopsy or cone biopsy results, when you are aware that a severe abnormality is apparent, is often a time of mixed emotion.

The results of your biopsy may take 7-10 days — a time of incredible anxiety and apprehension mixed with fear for your life if indeed cancer is found; fear of having to have a hysterectomy; as well as fear that you may no longer be able to have children.

When your results are available you will generally be notifed and an appointment made to discuss these results with your doctor. It is a good idea to take your partner, family member or trusted friend along with you, since they will not feel as upset and stressed as you and will be able to listen to the doctor with more objectivity.

If you find yourself in the position where you are told you have cancer of the cervix, your emotions are often mixed and varied. You may feel stunned and shocked with a sense of disbelief that this could happen to you. Until this moment of diagnosis you will still often cling to the hope that all will be well and cancer will not be found.

At this time, when you are told you have cervical cancer, there is absolutely every reason not to lose hope, because early cancer of the cervix can be **successfully treated**.

If, up to this time, you have been seeing a gynaecologist, once the diagnosis of cervical cancer has been confirmed, you should be referred to a gynaecologist-oncologist.

If, however, your gynaecologist recommends and intends to personally perform a hysterectomy on you, you might like to ask about their level of expertise in the field of cervical cancer. The clinical stage and type of cancer you have will determine which **type** of hysterectomy you have, or whether radiotherapy may be recommended prior to surgery.

Whilst you may feel uncomfortable in questioning your doctor's expertise in the treatment of cervical cancer, it is in your best interest to do so.   Often a sense of urgency may prevail in recommending immediate treatment and you will probably be eager to undergo this. Since the interval between diagnosis and a second opinion from a gynaecologist-oncologist may be a few weeks, do not feel concerned and worried that your cancer is "growing out of control" during this time.

This does **not** occur in a few weeks and in the best interest of your health and well-being, you should ask your gynaecologist for a referral to a gynaecologist-oncologist.

Having had a false negative Pap smear result three months earlier, my cervical cancer was discovered incidently during routine pathology analysis of my uterus and cervix, following a hysterectomy for another condition.

My gynaecologist **telephoned** me two weeks later to inform me of this and tried to reassure me that I was very lucky to have had the correct treatment. I was very shocked and upset and wondered if I should see a cancer specialist to make sure all was well.

After three days I rang my gynaecologist back and asked if I should see an oncologist. Giving, what I considered to be good reasons at the time, he dissuaded me.

I started to have a few nagging doubts and by now my anxieties had turned into a quest for the truth. I then sought the advice of my GP and was subsequently referred to a gynaecologist-oncologist. I was then readmitted to hospital and underwent a further six hours of surgery. My advice? **If in doubt always seek a second opinion.**

One Woman's Comments

The Role of the Gynaecologist-Oncologist

At my first visit to my gynaecologist-oncologist I went alone; as far as I was concerned it was purely for a second opinion. As he drew diagrams and explained the criteria for surgery, I remember thinking: "Gee, this is serious — I'm glad it's not going to happen to me".

It was half-way through the consultation when I realised he **was** talking about me! He then very calmly and patiently repeated it all again!

One Woman's Comments

A recognised gynaecologist-oncologist works solely in the field of **reproductive cancer**, giving you both the availability of experience and optimal treatment essential for the eradication of this disease.

Your gynaecologist-oncologist will explain the nature of cancer and should draw diagrams so you understand where your cancer is and the nature of your disease, as well as explaining treatment methods best suited to your "stage" of disease.

Treatment is not initiated until your cancer is "staged" and this is based on FIGO (Federation of International Gynaecology and Obstetrics 1986) guidelines for the treatment of cervical cancer. This method of assessment determines the exact location and spread of your disease, allowing the initiation of optimal treatment. Such an assessment is made by two gynaecologist-oncologists in consultation with a histo-pathologist who microscopically examines cancerous tissue. The life-threatening nature of invasive cancer mandates a team effort in cancer diagnosis and the appropriate treatment for your stage of cancer.

Treatment methods will vary and can range from a cone biopsy for micro-invasive cancer (where childbearing is of importance), to a simple hysterectomy where childbearing is not an issue. Other treatment methods for invasive cervical cancer require a radical hysterectomy, radiotherapy or chemotherapy — either alone or in combination — suitable to your stage and type of cancer.

Most gynaecologist-oncologists are very frank and honest and will generally tell you the expected outcome, with the latest scientific results on your stage and type of cancer and the effect your treatment will have in terms of cure — generally excellent in early invasive cervical cancer.

My gynaecologist referred me to a gynaecologist-oncologist for a second opinion. On that first visit to him, he drew diagrams and explained why I needed a radical hysterectomy, with helpful hints during and after hospitalisation, follow-up care and my expected prognosis in terms of cure. He treated me as an equal and suggested I ring him at any time before surgery if I had further questions — which I did.

I had a strong feeling that we were a team in this, and whilst shocked and stunned at my diagnosis, he will never know how close I came to hugging him at the sense of relief I felt at his humane and compassionate qualities, which were so evident in that first consultation with him.

One Woman's Comments

Types of Cervical Cancer

When cancer of the cervix has occurred, the name of the cancer refers to the cells from which the cancer originates. Cervical cancer may therefore be called—

- ### Squamous Cell Carcinoma
  Comprises 85% of all cervical cancers and originates from the squamous cells of the cervix (refer to Figure No 12).

- ### Adeno Carcinoma (carcinoma of the columnar cells)
  Comprises 10% of cervical cancers and originates from the columnar cells in the endocervical canal (refer to Figure No 13).

- ### Adeno-squamous Carcinoma
  Comprises 5% of cervical cancers where there are two types of cancer cells present — originating from the columnar cells and the squamous cells. This form of cancer is less common and mostly originates at the transformation zone.

Signs and Symptoms of Cervical Cancer

The presence of abnormal cells or pre-cancerous cells in the cervix, cause **no** signs or symptoms and can **only** be detected by a Pap smear test. If abnormal cells have progressed to an invasive cancer there are some physical symptoms which will occur—

- In early invasive cancer the first symptom may be an increase in vaginal discharge — usually watery and clear, but sometimes slightly bloodstained. Often this is dismissed by a woman, who may rationalise this as being due to her hormone levels or the normal increase of vaginal secretions during ovulation. However, for some women, the clear watery discharge is constant and obvious. Many women will not notice changes in their vaginal secretions at all.

- The blood supply to the cervix is abundant and as cancer cells invade further into the cervix and permeate the small blood vessels, abnormal spotting and irregular vaginal bleeding between periods will occur. Bleeding may occur after sexual intercourse and this may range from slight spotting to moderate dark blood loss.

- Some women may experience pain or discomfort during or after intercourse.

> Any woman who experiences bleeding after intercourse, bleeding after menopause or irregular bleeding between menstrual periods, should see her doctor for a Pap smear test and full investigation. Irrespective of the smear result it is highly likely that a colposcopic examination will be recommended.

"Stages" of Cervical Cancer

As we have already seen, before any treatment for cervical cancer can be commenced your cancer is "staged" to determine the exact location and spread of your disease.

There are four Stages of cervical cancer:

- **Stage I**   The cancer is confined to the cervix.

- **Stage II**   The cancer extends beyond the cervix.

- **Stage III**   The cancer extends to the pelvis and lower vagina.

- **Stage IV**   The cancer involves the pelvis, bladder or rectum and distant organs.

Since the treatment of cervical cancer is such a huge area to address, and has been covered in detail in my previous book *"Living for Tomorrow*—a positive approach to the treatment of cervical cancer", I have only included details on the "staging" of cervical cancer for added information.

Author's Note

Stage I

In Stage I the cancer is confined to the cervix and is further separated into—

• *Stage Ia*

Micro-invasive carcinoma.

— Stage Ia1

Minimal microscopic invasion — cancer cells have invaded up to 3mm beyond the basement membrane (see Figure 25).

— Stage Ia2

Lesions detected microscopically which can be measured — cancer cells have invaded up to 5mm beyond the basement membrane — the horizontal spread is no greater than 7mm — there may be capillary or lymph space involvement (see Figure 25).

• *Stage Ib*

Lesions of greater dimension than Stage Ia2 with capillary involvement — there may be lymph space involvement (see Figure 26).

Cancer "staging" is based on the FIGO (Federation of International Gynaecology and Obstetrics, 1986) method of assessment used to determine the exact location and spread of your disease, so that optimal treatment can be initiated.

Stage Ia

The risk of spread to pelvic lymph nodes is virtually nil in Stage Ia.

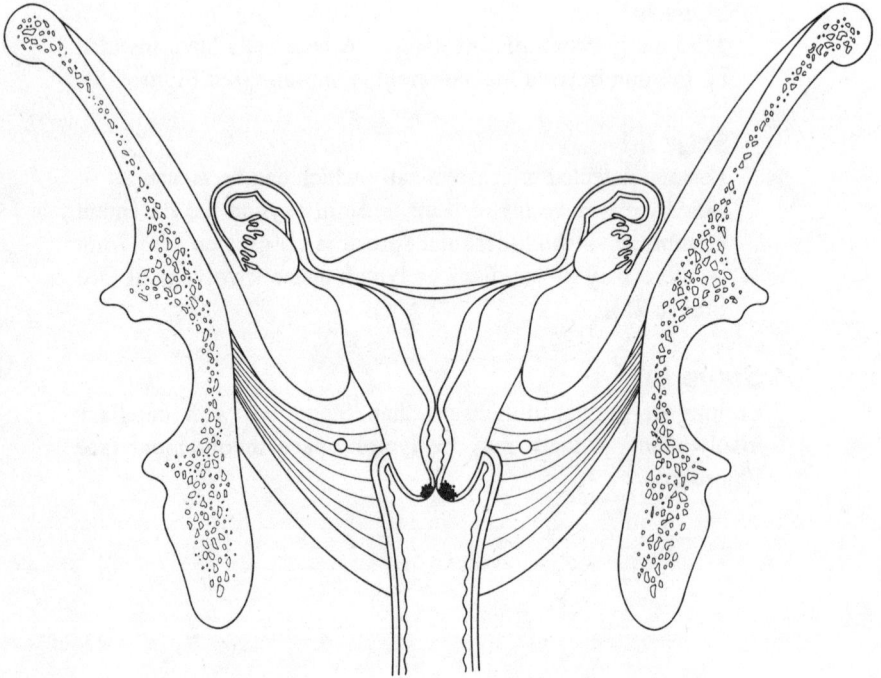

Figure 25—Cancer of the Cervix

Stage Ia1   **Stage Ia2**

Women diagnosed with these Stages of cancer usually present with an abnormal smear and the cancer is invisible to the naked eye.   Diagnosis will be made on colposcopic examination and cone biopsy

Stage Ib

Since the cancer has penetrated into the deeper tissues of the cervix, involving the capillaries and possibly lymph vessels, it is now classified as "invasive cancer' and has the capacity to spread to the pelvic lymph nodes.

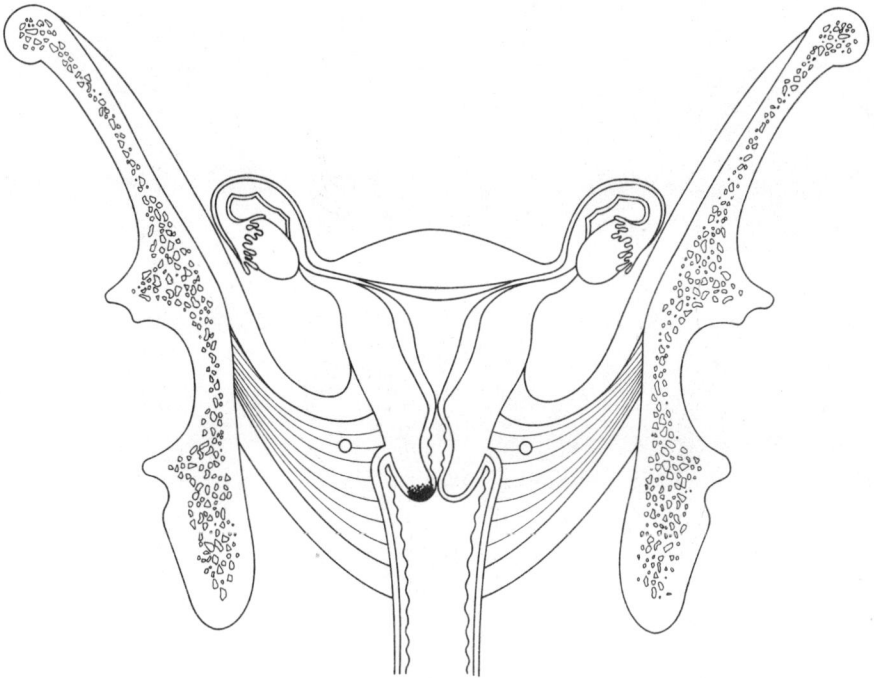

Figure 26—Cancer of the Cervix—Stage Ib
Invasive cancer of this nature has the ability to spread to the pelvic lymph nodes

Stages II — IV

For further detailed information on the methods of treatment for cervical cancer, including the emotional, physical, social and sexual implications of this disease, please refer to my first book, *"Living for Tomorrow*—a positive approach to the treatment of cervical cancer".

PART VI

Living for Tomorrow

During your journey through this book there is no doubt that the experience of receiving an abnormal Pap smear result can and does cause differing emotional feelings — and fears — which can impact on you and your relationship with others.

This book may also pose and answer many questions which are uppermost in your mind at this time. However, if at any time you feel you would like further discussion with your doctor on Pap smears and are unsure or unconfident in talking about issues which are important to you, why not take this book with you to refer to? After all, it has been written as a baseline for encouraging open, informed discussion between you and your doctor.

If at any time you have doubts or an uneasy feeling at any stage about an abnormal Pap smear result, or continuing abnormal symptoms, do take action — get a second opinion. If you are wrong, so what? No harm has been done. But if you are right, you will be forever thankful that you followed your intuition.

Margaret

P for *Plan*

Having a Pap smear test each year — or at the very least two-yearly — is imperative. If the State in which you live does not have a Pap Smear Registry which sends out reminder letters each two years, you can obtain a Pap Smear Reminder Card by ringing the toll free number 008 80 8725. The reminder card lasts for 10 years.

A for *Abnormal*

Since a Pap smear test is a screening test only, it cannot be relied upon to **make** a diagnosis. The presence of CIN of any degree requires referral to a gynaecologist for investigation. Abnormal cells of the cervix are invisible to the naked eye and cause no signs or symptoms.

P for *Persistence*

If your abnormal Pap smear result indicates CIN or you have abnormal symptoms with a negative Pap smear result, be persistent in requesting a referral to a gynaecologist for further investigation. Whilst many doctors **will** refer you, some will not. Be persistent in your efforts for a referral or alternatively see another GP for referral, or make an appointment at the dysplasia clinic of a women's hospital (listed at the end of this book).

S for **Self**

It is your individual responsibility to care for your health by utilising the preventative screening tests available. It is also your responsibility to obtain the results.

M for **Mother**

The incidence of cervical cancer increases with age and women over 50 are at the highest risk — most women in this age group have not had a Pap smear for many years. Ask your mother when she last had a Pap smear test, and next time you make an appointment to have yours, why not make one for her too — and take her with you.

E for **Embarrassment**

We often feel a little embarrassed having a Pap smear test. However, if abnormal cells are detected they can be simply and effectively treated **before** they progress to cervical cancer.

A for **Ask**

Clear understanding of abnormal cells of the cervix, and medical investigative procedures and treatment will often reduce your fears of the unknown. Ask questions of your doctor when you do not understand what is happening to you.

R for **Research**

No test is perfect and the Pap smear test is no exception. However, it is the **only** test we have for detecting abnormal cells of the cervix.

PART VII

Glossary

A

Acetic acid

A diluted solution of vinegar which when applied to the cervix, identifies abnormal areas

Adeno carcinoma (of the cervix)

Cancer of the columnar cells situated in the endocervical canal of the cervix

Adeno squamous carcinoma

Cancer of the squamous cells and columnar cells; generally originates at the transformation zone of the cervix

Ayres spatula

Type of wooden spatula used to take Pap smears of the cervix

B

Basement membrane

A membrane which separates the cervical epithelium (skin) from the underlying tissue of the cervix which contains capillary and lymphatic vessels

Biopsy, Cone

See **Cone biopsy**

Biopsy, Punch

See **Punch biopsy**

Body-image

Personal image of how we view our own body

C

Cancer

The growth of abnormal cells which are malignant and have the ability to multiply, destroying normal cells and tissue. Malignant cells also have the capacity to spread via the blood stream and lymphatic vessels and implant in other areas of the body and grow

Carcinoma

The technical medical term for cancer

Carcinoma insitu

Now known as CIN 3 (Severe Dysplasia), Carcinoma insitu is one of the Stages (grades) of pre-cancer of the cervix

Cautery
Cauterisation

Destruction of abnormal cells of the cervix via freezing or burning (diathermy)

Cell

A structural and functional unit which has the ability to grow and reproduce and from which tissue is formed. A cell contains a nucleus which is the important centre of growth and is surrounded by cytoplasm

Cervical Intra-
epithelial
Neoplasia

C = Cervix
I = Intra-epithelial [within the skin]
N = Neoplasia [change in the cells])

Abbreviated as CIN — abnormal cells of the cervix are classified according to the number of abnormal cells present

Cervix   The entrance to the uterus

CIN   See Cervical Intra-epithelial Neoplasia

Colposcope   A binocular microscope which
                            magnifies the cervix 8-30 times,
                            enabling the inspection of the vagina
                            and cervix

Colposcopic   The inspection of the cervix with a
examination   colposcope, which is used to identify
                            the location, size and area of abnormal
                            cells of the cervix

Columnar cells   Column-shaped cells which line the
                            endocervical canal of the cervix. The
                            cells produce mucus

Cone biopsy   The removal of a cone-shaped segment
                            of tissue from the cervix

Cryo-cautery   A method of destroying abnormal cells
Cry-surgery   of the cervix by treating them with a
                            freezing technique using carbon dioxide
                            or nitrous oxide

Cytobrush   Similar in appearance to a cosmetic
                            mascara brush, the cytobrush may be
                            used to take a sample of cells from the
                            endocervical canal when taking a Pap
                            smear

Cytology   The study of cells

Cytologist   A person specialising in the study of
                            cells

D

Diathermy

The use of an electric current to produce heat in underlying tissues which may be used to treat abnormal cells of the cervix

Dysplasia

See CIN

E

Ectocervix

The surface of the cervix and external OS where it encroaches into the vagina

Endocervical canal

The canal leading from the cervix to the uterus

Endocervical cells

Columnar cells which line the endocervical canal

Endocervical glands

Mucus-producing glands which line the endocervical canal

Epithelium

Medical terminology for skin

External OS

The entrance to the endocervical canal

F

False negative

A Pap smear or colposcopy result which mistakenly reports that there are no abnormal cells of the cervix

False positive   A Pap smear or colposcopy result which mistakenly reports the existence of abnormal cells

Female re-productive organs   These comprise the uterus (womb), fallopian tubes, ovaries, cervix and vagina — all situated in the pelvic area

G

Genital warts   Caused by the Human Papilloma Virus and resulting in the presence of small warts on a woman's cervix, vagina or vulva and on a man's penis

General Practitioner   (GP) A family doctor who cares for your general health

Gynaecologist   A doctor whose field of expertise is the diagnosis, care and treatment of reproductive disorders and diseases in women

Gynaecologist-Obstetrician   The same as a gynaecologist, but also possess expertise in the care of women during pregnancy and birth

Gynaecologist-Oncologist   The same as a gynaecologist, but also has expertise in the diagnosis, management and treatment of women with cancer located in their reproductive organs

H

Hormone

A chemical released by glands in some areas of the body. The ovaries produce the female hormones oestrogen and progesterone

Human Papilloma Virus

(HPV) (Wart Virus) Caused by the Human Papilloma Virus and sometimes resulting in the presence of small warts on a woman's cervix, vagina or vulva and on a man's penis. For many women the presence of HPV causes no symptoms and will be detected on Pap smear only. HPV may cause some microscopic changes to the cells of the cervix, which **may** progress to CIN in some women. Also see Genital warts

Hysterectomy— Simple

The surgical removal of the uterus and cervix. Sometimes the fallopian tubes and the ovaries are removed as well

Hysterectomy— Radical (Wertheim's)

The surgical removal of the uterus, cervix, upper third of the vagina, fallopian tubes, pelvic ligaments and tissues which support the uterus, pelvic lymph nodes and sometimes the ovaries in the treatment of invasive cervical cancer

I

Invasive cervical cancer   Cancer cells invading through the basement membrane, the blood vessels and lymphatic vessels of the cervix

L

Langerhans cells   Local defence cells present in the cervix

Libido   An individual's desire for sexual expression

Lymphocytes   White blood cells which help combat infection

M

Malignant   Abnormal cells which are able to multiply, grow and spread to other tissues and organs in an uncontrolled manner. If not removed they will result in death

Metastasis   Transfer of malignant cells via blood and lymphatic vessels to other organs where they implant and grow, invading tissues, blood vessels, lymphatics and organs

Micro-invasive cancer	Malignant cells which have broken through the basement membrane of the cervix to a depth of up to 3mm
Menstruation	Cyclical (approximately every 28 days) bleeding from the uterus when pregnancy has not occurred
Metaplasia	Normal physiological changing of columnar cells into squamous cells at the transformation zone

N

Normal Pap smear	A Pap smear test which reveals no abnormalities of the cells of the cervix, the endocervical canal or the transformation zone
Nucleus	The growth centre of a cell

O

OS—internal	The opening at the top of the endocervical canal into the uterus
OS—external	The entrance to the endocervical canal of the cervix
Oestrogen	A hormone produced by the ovaries

P

Papanicolaou, George Nicholaus (1889-1962)	Developed the Pap smear test in the 1920s
Pap smear test	A test developed by George Nicholaus Papanicolaou in the 1920s which is a screening test to detect abnormal cells of the cervix
Polar Probe	This probe, which will be used to detect abnormal tissue of the cervix, is currently undergoing clinical trials
Progesterone	A hormone produced by the ovaries
Punch biopsy	A punch biopsy is a test which involves the taking of very tiny samples of abnormal cells of the cervix observed at colposcopic examination

R

Radical hysterectomy	See Hysterectomy—radical
Radiotherapy	The treatment of a disease by the use of radiation which may be ionising radiation, radium or radioactive substances

S

Simple hysterectomy

See Hysterectomy—simple

Speculum

An instrument which, when inserted, separates the walls of the vagina, enabling observation of the cervix

Squamo columnar junction

See transformation zone

Squamous cells

This is the name given to the cells which line the vagina and outer surface of the cervix

Squamous cell carcinoma

The growth of malignant or cancerous cells arising from squamous cells

Stage of cancer

A method of assessment based on the FIGO (Federation of International Gynaecology and Obstetrics 1986) standards which determine the exact location and spread of cervical cancer

Staging

The extent of the cancer which is characterised by clinical findings and pathology analysis of tissue

Stenosis

A constriction or narrowing

T

Transformation zone

This is the area of the cervix, also called the squamo-columnar junction, where the columnar cells change into squamous cells and this changing of cells is normal and called metaplasia

Tumour, malignant

The growth of abnormal malignant cells arising from normal tissue

U

Uterus

Also known as the womb, the uterus is a muscular structure where an embryo implants and grows into a foetus for 40 weeks

V

Vagina

Also known as the birth canal, the vagina is a canal leading from the external genitals to the cervix and uterus

Virus

A minute micro-organism which infects humans and is totally dependent on living cells for reproduction

W

Wertheim's radical hysterectomy

See Hysterectomy, radical

Index

A

B

C

129

F

G

H

I

L

S

T

U

V

W

Bibliography

BAIRD PJ, 1985 *Cervical Cancer and the Papanicolaou Smear*, Australian Family Physician, Volume 14, pp 543-544.

BIRNBAUER B, 1994 *Pap Screening Labs Face Legal Crisis*, The Age, Friday 8 April, p 1.

BUCKLEY JD 1981 *et al, Case Control Study of the Husbands of Women with Dysplasia or Carcinoma of the Cervix Uteri*, Lancet 2, pp 1110-14.

CAMPION MJ, BROWN JR, McCANCE DJ, ATIA W, EDWARDS R, CUZICK J, and SINGER A, 1988 *Psychosexual Trauma of an Abnormal Cervical Smear*, British Journal of Obstetrics and Gynaecology, Vol 95, pp 175-181.

DUNCAN I, 1988 *Update Advances in the Prevention and Treatment of Gynaecological Malignancy*, from the Post Graduate Centres, pp 30-31.

GRANT P, BEISCHER N, PLANNER R, 1992 *The Treatment of Gynaecological Malignancy in a General Public Hospital*, The Medical Journal of Australia, Volume 157, p 380.

LEWIS D, MITCHELL H, 1994, *An Evaluation of Cervical Screening in General Practice*, The Medical Journal of Australia, Vol 160, pp 628-632.

MAKAY E, BEISCHER N, PEPPERELL R, WOOD C, 1992 *Illustrated Textbook of Gynaecology*, 2nd Edition, WB Saunders Bailliére Tindall, Figure 35.6, Photograph of Instruments for Cervical Smear courtesy of Professor N Beischer, University of Melbourne.

MAKAY E, BEISCHER N, PEPPERELL R, WOOD C, 1992 *Illustrated Textbook of Gynaecology*, 2nd Edition, WB Saunders Bailliére Tindall, pp 467-499.

McDONALD TW, NEUTENS JJ, FISCHER L, JESSEE D, 1989 *Impact of Cervical Intraepithelial Neoplasia Diagnosis and Treatment on Self-esteem and Body Image*, Gynaecologic Oncology, Vol 34, pp 345-349.

MITCHELL H, 1990 *Epidemiology of Cervical Cancer and Screening*, Australian Cancer Society, Cancer Forum 14, No 3, pp 143-154.

MITCHELL H, HIGGINS V, 1990-1993 *Victorian Cervical Cytology Registry Statistical Reports*.

PLANNER R, University of Melbourne, Department of Gynaecology-Oncology, Mercy Hospital for Women, Melbourne, Figures 19 and 20.

QUINN M, 1990 *Management of Women with Cytological Abnormalities on Pap Smear*, Australian Cancer Society, Cancer Forum 14, No 3, pp 155-159.

RICHARDSON AC, LYON JB, 1981 *The Effect of Condom Use on Squamous Cell Cervical Intraepithelial Neoplasia*, American Journal of Obstetrics and Gynaecology, pp 909-913.

ROSE R, 1983 *Cervical Cancer*, Australian Family Physician, Volume 12, No 11, pp 778-81.

SIMONS A, PHILLIPS D, COLEMAN D, 1993 *Damage to D.N.A. in Cervical Epithelium Related to Smoking Tobacco*, British Medical Journal, Volume 306, p 1444.

SHIPES E, 1987 *Nursing Clinics of North America*, Psychosocial Issues: The Person with an Ostomy, Vol 22, No 2, pp 292-93.

SKLADNEV V, CEO, *Polartechnics*, Sydney, Australia, research into Polar probe.

STAFL A, KOLSTADT P, 1982 *The Atlas of Colposcopy*, 3rd Edition, Churchill Livingston, Figure 46 reproduced courtesy of Professor A Stafl.

THE ROYAL AUSTRALIAN COLLEGE OF OBSTETRICIANS AND GYNAECOLOGISTS 1991, *Screening for the Prevention of Cervical Cancer*, Policy No 13, p 1.

THOMAS I, WRIGHT G, WARD B 1990, *The Effect of Condom Use on Cervical Intraepithelial Neoplasia Grade 1 [CIN 1]*, Australia & New Zealand Journal of Obstetrics and Gynaecology, pp 30-32, 236-239.

WARD J, SANSON FISHER RW, 1990 *Cervical Cancer Screening in General Practice: Standards of Care, Barriers and Strategies for Change*, Australian Cancer Society, Cancer Forum 14, No 3, pp 150-152.

WILSON M, PLANNER R, 1993 *Psychosexual Consequences of Gynaecological Malignancy in Young Women Following Wertheim's Radical Hysterectomy*, Paper presented to National Conference of Psychosomatic Obstetrics and Gynaecology, August 1993.

1986 *Federation of International Gynaecology Obstetrics*, Staging of Cervical Cancer.

Organisations

The following hospitals and organisations provide advice on services related to health care, abnormal Pap smears and cervical cancer. These names and addresses are included for readers' information as a reference point for those who are interested. They are not to be read as inferring any sponsorship, approval or affiliation of either the author or this publication.

Schedules are not intended to be exhaustive and readers should make their own enquires of these institutions and organisations and others for further information of the services and facilities available.

These details are provided in good faith for the information of interested persons and are based on enquires made in August 1993. The hospitals and organisations provide advice or services of a gynaecological-oncology nature.

Hospitals

VICTORIA
Mercy Hospital for Women
126 Clarendon Street
East Melbourne 3002
Phone (03) 270 2222

Royal Womens Hospital
132 Grattan Street
Carlton 3053
Phone (03) 344 2000

Monash Medical Centre
246 Clayton Road
Clayton 3168
Phone (03) 550 1111

NEW SOUTH WALES
Royal Prince Alfred Hospital
Missenden Road
Camperdown 2050
Phone (02) 516 6111

Westmead Hospital
Darcy Road
Westmead 2145
Phone (02) 633 6333

King George V Hospital
Missendon Road
Camperdown 2050
Phone (02) 516 6111

NEW SOUTH WALES (Cont'd)
Royal North Shore Hospital
Pacific Highway
St Leonards 2065
Phone (02) 438 7111

Royal Hospital for Women
118 Oxford Street
Paddington 2021
Phone (02) 339 4111

SOUTH AUSTRALIA
Royal Adelaide Hospital
North Terrace
Adelaide 5000
Phone (08) 223 0230

Queen Elizabeth Hospital
28 Woodville Road
Woodville South 5011
Phone (08) 345 0222

TASMANIA
Queen Alexander Hospital
Liverpool Street
Hobart 7000
Phone (002) 38 8308

QUEENSLAND
Mater Hospital
Raymond Terrace
South Brisbane 4101
Phone (07) 840 8111

Royal Womens Hospital
Bowen Bridge Road
Herston 4029
Phone (07) 253 8111

WESTERN AUSTRALIA
King Edward Memorial Hospital
Bagot Road
Subiaco 6008
Phone (09) 340 2222

Member Organisations of the Australian Cancer Society Inc

AUSTRALIAN CAPITAL TERRITORY
ACT Cancer Society
PO Box 316
Curtin ACT 2605
Phone (06) 285 3070

VICTORIA
Anti-Cancer Council of Victoria
1 Rathdowne Street
Carlton South 3053
Phone (03) 279 1111

SOUTH AUSTRALIA
Anti-Cancer Foundation of the
Universities of South Australia
North Adelaide 5006
Phone (08) 267 5222

QUEENSLAND
Queensland Cancer Fund
PO Box 201
Spring Hill 4000
Phone (07) 257 1155

WESTERN AUSTRALIA
Cancer Foundation of WA
42 Ord Street
West Perth 6005
Phone (09) 321 6224

NEW SOUTH WALES
NSW State Cancer Council
GPO Box 7070
Sydney 2001
Phone (02) 264 8888

NORTHERN TERRITORY
Northern Territory Anti-Cancer
Foundation
PO Box 42719
Casuarina 0811
Phone (089) 27 4888

TASMANIA
Tasmanian Cancer Committee
GPO Box 191B
Hobart 7001
Phone (002) 35 4895

Gynaecological Cancer Support Groups

Victoria
Cervical Cancer Support Group
Bronwyn (03) 754 2803

Tasmania
Gynaecological Cancer Support
Group
GPO Box 2739
Hobart 7001
Phone (002) 44 3030
(Co-ordinator)

Miscellaneous

Victorian Cervical Cytology Registry
PO Box 61
Carlton south 3053
Phone (03) 349 1799

Women's Health Program
Cliveden Hill Private Hospital
29 Simpson Street
East Melbourne 3002
Phone (03) 419 7122
Women's Health Co-ordinator or
Director of Nursing